Study Guide for Leifer

THOMPSON'S INTRODUCTION TO MATERNITY AND PEDIATRIC NURSING

Third Edition

Jean Weiler Ashwill, MSN, RN, CPNP
Director, Center for Continuing Nursing Education
Univeristy of Texas at Arlington School of Nursing
Arlington, Texas

Emily Slone McKinney, MSN, RNC
Education Coordinator
Women's & Children's Services
Baylor Medical Center at Irving
Irving, Texas

W.B. Saunders Company
A Division of Harcourt Brace & Company
Philadelphia London Toronto Montreal Sydney Tokyo

W.B. SAUNDERS COMPANY
A Division of Harcourt Brace & Company
Independence Square West
Philadelphia, PA 19106

Study Guide for Leifer
THOMPSON'S INTRODUCTION TO
MATERNITY AND PEDIATRIC NURSING,
Third Edition

ISBN 0–7216–8018–6

Printed in the United States of America.

Last digit is the print number: 9 8 7 6 5 4 3 2 1

Preface

This Study Guide is written to promote student mastery of *Thompson's Introduction to Maternity and Pediatric Nursing,* Third Edition, by Gloria Leifer. Each chapter in this Study Guide corresponds to the text chapter having the same number and title.

The authors have included matching and completion **Learning Activities** to help students learn basic factual knowledge that underlies nursing care. Other exercises request the student to list or describe text information to encourage reading comprehension and written expression of what is learned. Labeling of illustrations is included to help the student understand anatomy, as appropriate.

To promote higher level learning, the authors have included **Thinking Critically,** which asks the student to apply knowledge or draw conclusions based on material in the textbook but not directly answered in the textbook. **Case Studies** and **Other Learning Activities** provide ideas for applying factual content to client care.

Each chapter concludes with multiple choice **Review Questions.** The questions ask for appropriate nursing actions, what the nurse should expect in terms of medical orders or usual care of the client and what complication the client is at risk of developing, as well as items that review basic factual information from the chapter.

An **Answer Key** for the Learning Activities and Review Questions is provided in the *Instructor's Manual for Thompson's Introduction to Maternity and Pediatric Nursing,* Third Edition. Rationales are included with the answers to the Review Questions.

Contents

Student Name 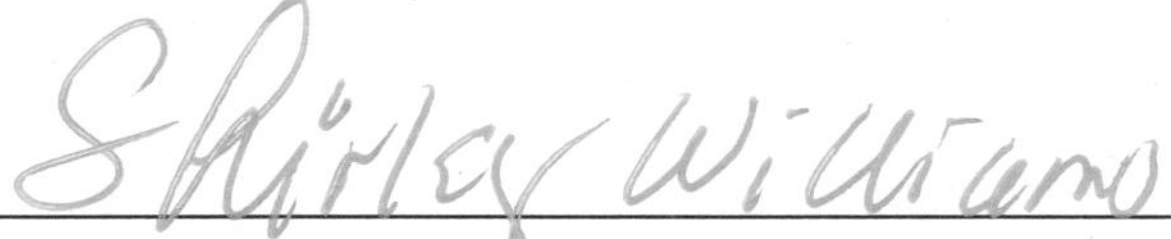

chapter **1**

The Past, the Present, and the Future of Maternity and Pediatric Nursing

LEARNING ACTIVITIES

1. Match the terms in the left column with their definitions on the right (a–e).

- A certified nurse-midwife (CNM)
- D clinical pathways
- E Diagnosis Related Group (DRG)
- C family-centered care
- B variance

a. a registered nurse with advanced training and certification in the care of women during pregnancy, birth, and the postpartum period

b. the difference between expected outcome and the outcome achieved

c. recognizing the strength and integrity of the family as the core of planning and implementing health care

d. collaborative guidelines for care within a time line

e. determination of hospital payment based on a patient's diagnosis

2. List three health-care professionals who deliver babies.

a. Obstetrician

b. Certified Nurse-Midwife

c. Obstetric

3. Match the names in the left column with their contributions toward improvement of maternal, newborn, and pediatric care on the right (a–j).

H Soranus
D Karl Credé
E Ignaz Semmelweis
B Louis Pasteur
G Joseph Lister
F Samuel Bard
A Oliver Wendell Holmes
I Abraham Jacobi
J Margaret Sanger
C Lillian Wald

a. associated dissection of cadavers by medical students and the incidence of puerperal fever among postpartum women

b. determined that puerperal fever was caused by bacteria that could be spread by people and objects

c. helped establish the Children's Bureau, leading to birth registration in all states and school lunch programs

d. developed a treatment to prevent blindness caused by gonorrhea

e. wrote a paper about contagiousness of puerperal fever

f. wrote the first American textbook on obstetrics

g. applied antiseptic principles to surgical practice

h. introduced podalic version to deliver the second twin

i. established pediatric nursing as a separate specialty

j. provided care for poor pregnant women

4. List three professional organizations concerned with maternity nursing.

a. The American College of Nurse Midwife (AC[illegible]

b. Assoc. of Women Health Obstet. Neo. Nurse (AWHON[illegible]

c. Nurse Assoc. of the Amer. College of Obstet. & Gynecol (NAACOG)

5. How has pediatric care in hospitals changed since the 1960s?

By the 60's a separate pediatric unit in hospital. However parents were restricted by rigid visiting hours that allowed parent infant contact for only a few hours each day.

Student Name Shirley Williams

6. Describe how each listed governmental program influences maternity and pediatric care.

   a. Title V amendment of the Public Health Services Act

   Title V amendment of Public Health Service act established Maternal-Infant Care Centers in public clinics.

   b. Title XIX of the Medicaid program

   Title XIX of the Medicaid program increases access to care by indigent women.

   c. Head Start program

   Head start programs were established to increase educational exposure of preschool children.

   d. National Center for Family Planning

   The National Center for Family Planning provides conceptive information.

   e. Women's, Infant's and Children's program

   (WIC) Program provides supplemental food + education for the poor

   f. Fair Labor Standards Act

   Passed in 1938, estab. a general min. working age of 16 + min. working age of 18 for jobs considered Hazardous.

   g. White House conferences

   Lists 17 statements related to the needs of children in the areas of education, health, welfare, + protection. This declaration has been widely distributed thru out the world.

7. How has the hospital stay for birth changed recently? What implication do these changes have for nurses?

8. How have consumers changed practices in maternity care?

In the Early 1960's the natural childbirth movement awakened expectant parents to the need for education + involvement.

9. How have advances in technology contributed to the growing population of chronically ill children?

High-risk perinatal clinics + neonatal intensive care unit enable 1-lb preemie to survive. Children c̄ ♡ problem are now treated by pediatric cardiologist

10. Describe the following methods of health-care financing.

a. HMO

Serves the more financially stable people (private insurance.)

b. PPO

Serves the less financially stable people (Medicare + Medicaid.)

11. Give two examples of advanced practice nurses.

a. PNP - Pediatric Nurse Practitioner

b. CNS - Clinical Nurse Specialists

12. List the steps of the nursing process.

a. Assessment

b. Analysis

c. Planning

d. Outcome identification

e. Implementation

f. Evaluation

13. What is *Healthy People 2000*?

is a national health promotion that is a vision for the new century

Student Name Shirley Williams S.P.N.

14. Describe each type of alternative therapy listed below. State any specific risks involved with the therapy.

    a. Osteopathy

    Combine manipulative therapy c̄ traditional (allopathic) medicine. Base on the theory that certain areas of the body are connected to specific identified pressure point on feet, hands, ears & others.

    b. Energy healing

    Involves the belief that an electromagnetic flow emerges from the therapist's hands & channel energy into the pt.

    c. Homeopathy

    Homeopathy uses plants, herbs & earth minerals that are thought to stimulate the body's immune system to deal c̄ specific health problems.

OTHER LEARNING ACTIVITIES

1. What is the typical hospital stay for a woman who has an uncomplicated vaginal birth at your clinical facility? For a woman who has an uncomplicated cesarean birth? Have any state laws affected length of stay? Ask nurses how they have changed their care to accommodate short postpartum hospital stays.

2. Talk with a father who was present at the birth of his child. How did the experience affect him? If he has more than one child and was not present at all the births, does he perceive any differences in how he feels toward his children based on whether he was present at their births?

3. When you are in the clinical area, care for a childbearing family from a cultural group other than your own. Use the assessment questions listed under "Cross-Cultural Considerations" in your text to better understand the family's views toward birth.

4. When you are in the clinical area, observe how the family is involved in the birth process. How do grandparents feel about the current trends in childbirth? How do you feel about the involvement of fathers in childbirth? Do you think siblings of the new baby should be involved? If so, in what way?

5. Ask the birth facility in your clinical area what types of statistical data they gather and what is done with that data.

6. Does your clinical facility use computerized charting in any way? What security measures are used for this type of charting?

REVIEW QUESTIONS

1. The Credé method prevents newborn eye infection by use of
   a. antibiotic ointment.
   b. silver nitrate solution.
   c. washing each eye separately.
   d. using gloves for all care.

2. The most important nursing action to prevent infection in any client is to
   a. use disposable equipment.
   b. consistently wash hands.
   c. limit visitors to family.
   d. wear hospital-laundered clothes.

3. To best improve the care of a pregnant woman from a different cultural group, the nurse should
   a. identify her expectations about pregnancy and birth.
   b. observe the woman and her family as they interact.
   c. learn about different local cultural groups.
   d. encourage her to adopt local childbearing practices.

4. Maternity or pediatric nurses may use statistics to
   a. determine daily staffing needs in hospitals.
   b. evaluate the outcomes of care given.
   c. predict the hospital census for the following year.
   d. compute the number of women who conceive each year.

5. In comparison to other developed countries, the United States' infant mortality rate is
   a. similar to developing nations.
   b. rapidly declining since 1990.
   c. higher than most European countries.
   d. lower than most European countries.

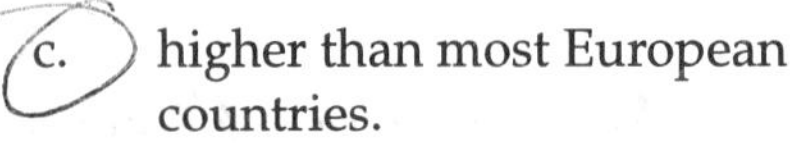

6. Choose the best description of certified nurse-midwife (CNM) qualifications.
   a. Attends uncomplicated births of low-risk women.
   b. Supervises prenatal care of high-risk women.
   c. Provides care to low-income women only.
   d. Gives limited care to women after normal childbirth.

7. The nursing process can best be described as a method to
   a. identify clients who have an increased risk for medical complications.
   b. reduce the incidence of complications for expectant mothers and infants.
   c. identify and solve client problems within the scope of nursing practice.
   d. promote breastfeeding in groups that do not usually nurse infants.

8. A variance in a clinical pathway means that
   a. the client did not cooperate with the therapy recommended.
   b. the outcome achieved differs from the expected outcome.
   c. care is individualized, appropriate to specific clients.
   d. limited reimbursement requires curtailment of health-care costs.

Student Name Shirley Williams S.P.N.

chapter **2**

Human Reproductive Anatomy and Physiology

LEARNING ACTIVITIES

1. Puberty is the time when reproductive systems mature and become capable of reproduction.

2. Boys begin outward changes of puberty between the ages of 10 and 13 years with growth of their penis and testes.

3. The first outward change of puberty in girls is Breast and occurs between the ages of 10 and 11 years.

4. Describe secondary sexual characteristics in boys and girls.

   a. Boys Pubic, axillary, chest & facial hair. Nocturnal Emissions & voice deepens.

   b. Girls hips broaden, Pubic & axillary hair appear.

5. Match the terms in the left column with their definitions on the right (a–h).

C androgens
F penis
H scrotum
B semen
G spermatogenesis
E spermatozoa
A testes
D testosterone

a. organs that produce spermatozoa and male sex hormones
b. seminal plasma plus sperm
c. male sex hormones
d. most abundant male hormone
e. male germ (reproductive) cells
f. male organ for urination and sexual intercourse
g. production of spermatozoa
h. skin sac that suspends testes away from the body

6. Label the structures of the male reproductive system on the figure below.

a. bladder
b. glans penis
c. penis
d. scrotum
e. testis
f. urethra
g. vas deferens

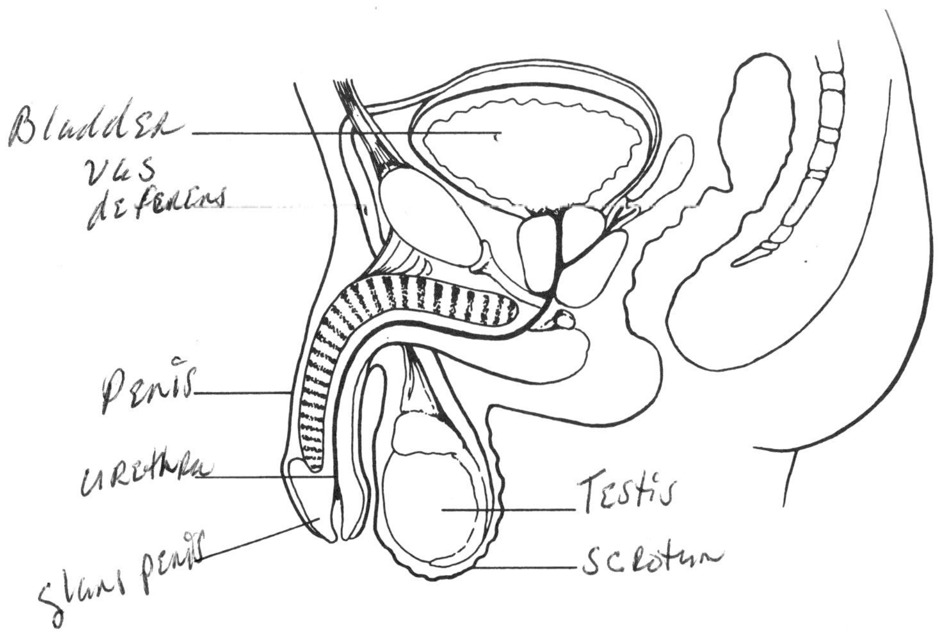

Student Name Shirley Williams S.P.N.

7. a. Spermatozoa are produced in the ______________ of the testes.

   b. Testosterone is produced in the Leydig cells of the testes.

8. Describe four effects of testosterone.

   a. increase muscle mass
   b. Promotes strength
   c. Promotes growth of long bones
   d. Enhances production of red blood cells

9. Label the structures of the internal female reproductive organs on the two figures below. Labels may be used more than once.

   a. bladder
   b. external os
   c. fallopian tube
   d. internal os
   e. ovary
   f. rectum
   g. urethra
   h. uterine fundus
   i. uterine cervix
   j. vagina

Fallopian tube
Uterine fundus
Bladder
Urethra
Fallopian tube
uterine cervix
rectum
Vagina

uterine fundus
fallopian tube
ovary
internal os
external os
Vagina
uterine cervix

10. Label the structures of the external female genitalia on the figure below.

a. clitoris
b. labia minora
c. labia majora
d. mons pubis
e. perineum
f. urethral opening
g. vaginal introitus

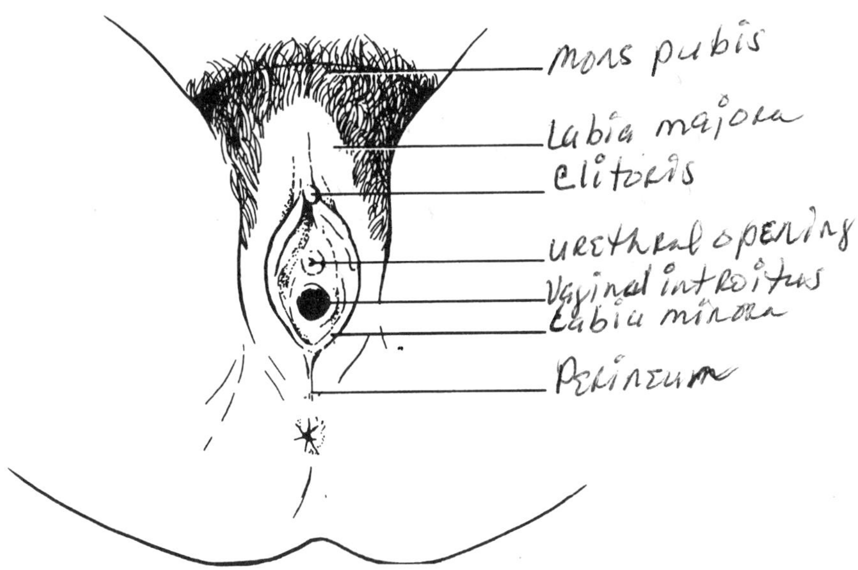

11. Match the female reproductive organs with their functions (a–k).

G Bartholin's glands
E cervical mucous membrane
D clitoris
C endometrium
H fallopian tubes
J myometrium
I ovaries
F rugae
K Skene's ducts
A uterus
B vagina

a. holds fetus during pregnancy
b. female organ of intercourse; passage for menstrual flow and fetus
c. uterine layer that responds to hormone changes during the menstrual cycle
d. small, sensitive erectile body
e. produces mucous plug during pregnancy
f. folds that permit vaginal distention during birth
g. produce lubrication of vagina during sexual arousal
h. usual location of fertilization
i. produce ova (female germ cells) and female hormones
j. muscular uterine layer to expel fetus at birth
k. lubricate urethra

Student Name Shirley Williams

12. Label each part of the female pelvis on the figure below.

a. coccyx
b. ischial spine
c. ischium
d. sacrum
e. symphysis pubis

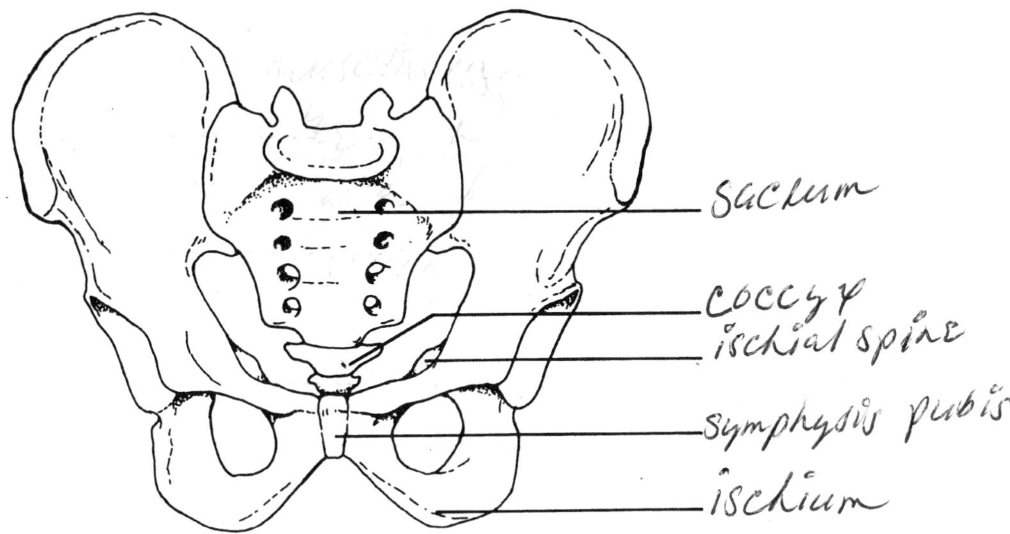

13. Label the following diameters of the pelvic inlet on the figure below and give the normal measurements for each.

a. anteroposterior
b. transverse
c. left oblique
d. right oblique

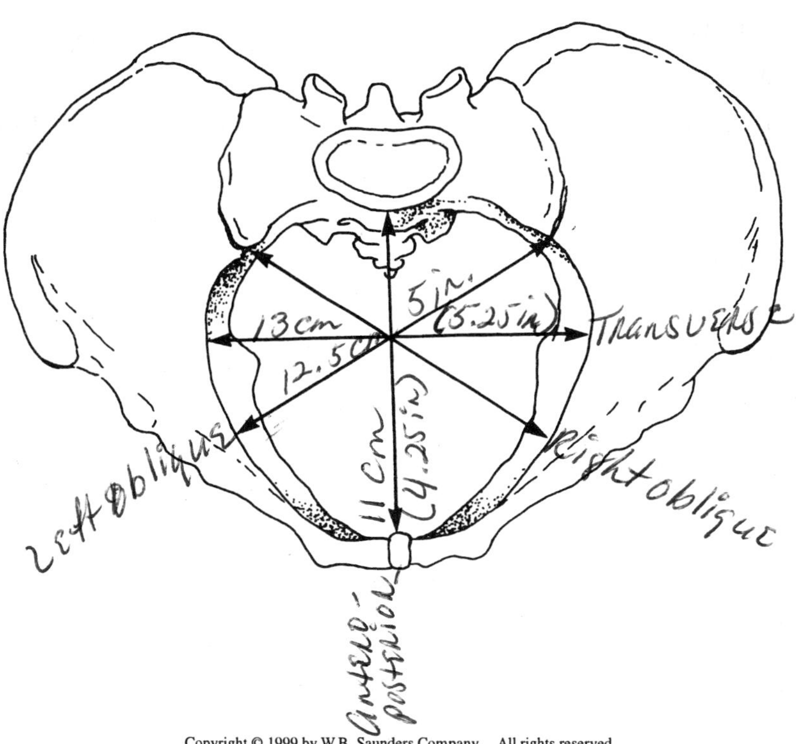

14. Label the structures of the female breast on the figure below.

a. nipple
b. areola
c. milk glands
d. lactiferous ducts

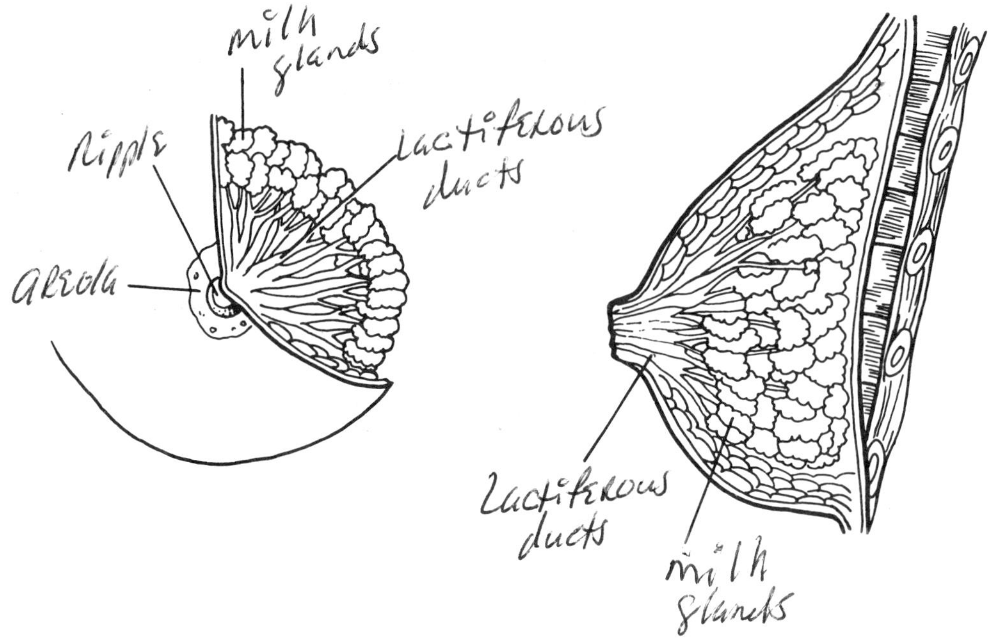

15. Match the female breast structures with their functions on the right (a–e).

B alveoli
E Cooper's ligaments
C lactiferous ducts
A lactiferous sinuses
D Montgomery's glands

a. widened area of a duct that holds milk
b. glands that secrete milk
c. carry milk from alveoli to nipple
d. secrete substance to protect breast during lactation
e. provide support for breast

16. Match the terms with their definitions on the right (a–g).

C corpus luteum
A dyspareunia
D menarche
B oogenesis
F ovarian follicle
E ovulation
G ovum

a. painful sexual intercourse
b. formation and development of an ovum
c. empty follicle after ovulation
d. first menstrual period
e. release of mature ovum
f. cavity containing a single ovum
g. female germ cell

Student Name Shirley Williams S.P.N.

17. State where each of the following female hormones is secreted and its function.

    a. FSH (follicle stimulating hormone)

    The anterior pituitary gland, FSH stimulates maturation of a follicle, a spherical cavity on an ovary that contains a single ovum.

    b. LH (luteinizing hormone)

    The anterior pituitary gland. LH stimulates final maturation & the release of an ovum

    c. Estrogen and progesterone

    Corpus luteum 12 days after ovulation, if fertilization has not occurred & progesterone & estrogen levels ↓. The fall in estrogen & progesterone causes the endometrium to break down resulting in menstruation.

THINKING CRITICALLY

1. Your 12-year-old niece confides to you that she is worried because she had her first menstrual period two months ago but has not had another one. She tells you she learned that most girls have periods once each month. What should you tell her?

2. Why might frequent douching cause problems such as vaginal infection?

OTHER LEARNING ACTIVITIES

1. Examine a model of the female pelvis. Identify the following landmarks.

    a. coccyx

    b. sacrum

    c. ischial spine

    d. symphysis pubis

    e. ilium

    f. linea terminalis

2. Identify the following pelvic diameters on a model of the female pelvis. Also, which diameter is the smallest in the inlet and outlet?

    Inlet:

    a. anteroposterior

    b. left and right oblique

    c. transverse

Cavity:

a. interspinous transverse

Outlet:

a. anteroposterior

b. intertuberous transverse

c. anterior-posterior sagittal

REVIEW QUESTIONS

1. At age 11 years, girls are often taller than boys because
   a. girls have higher levels of testosterone.
   b. boys begin puberty at an earlier age.
   c. girls begin puberty at an earlier age.
   d. girls have a higher hematocrit.

2. A woman can become pregnant even if the male "pulls out" before ejaculation because
   a. ejaculation occurs before insertion of the penis.
   b. some semen is released before ejaculation.
   c. sperm are added to semen after ejaculation.
   d. semen enters the vagina when the penis is inserted.

3. A woman comes to the clinic for a yearly check-up pelvic exam. She asks if it is all right for her to use a douche occasionally. The nurse should teach her that douching
   a. is unnecessary, but will do no harm.
   b. may hinder her vagina's natural cleansing action.
   c. adds to the natural cleansing action of her vagina.
   d. should never be done.

4. The ______ is the uterine layer that functions during labor to expel the fetus.
   a. parametrium
   b. myometrium
   c. endometrium

5. The ______ is the layer of the uterus that responds to cyclic hormonal changes of the menstrual cycle.
   a. parametrium
   b. myometrium
   c. endometrium

6. The typical pelvic type for a male is the
   a. android.
   b. anthropoid.
   c. gynecoid.
   d. platypelloid.

7. The ideal pelvic type for a female is the
   a. android.
   b. anthropoid.
   c. gynecoid.
   d. platypelloid.

8. Which division of the female pelvis can change slightly to accommodate the fetus during birth?
   a. pelvic inlet
   b. pelvic cavity
   c. pelvic outlet

Student Name Shirley Williams S.P.N.

9. Males are generally stronger than females at maturity because
   a. they begin puberty at an earlier age than females.
   b. testosterone promotes growth of a male's muscles.
   c. females start puberty at a later age than males.
   d. high estrogen production promotes bone growth.

10. The function of a male's scrotum is to
    a. regulate the temperature of the testes.
    b. carry sperm from the testes to the penis.
    c. secrete the hormone testosterone.
    d. increase the strength of ejaculation of sperm.

11. The breast structures that secrete milk after childbirth are the
    a. lactiferous ducts.
    b. Montgomery's glands.
    c. alveoli.
    d. nipples.

12. Erection of the penis occurs during sexual stimulation because
    a. strong muscles attached to the pelvis lift the penis.
    b. blood is trapped within the tissues of the organ.
    c. the testosterone level falls in response to stimulation.
    d. prostate gland secretions cause the organ to stiffen.

13. A woman's ova (egg cells) are formed
    a. from puberty to the last menstrual period.
    b. only during development before birth.
    c. by the dense outer layer of the ovary.
    d. within the distal fimbriae of the fallopian tube.

14. The middle muscular layer of the uterus has __A__ fibers.
    a. circular
    b. figure-eight
    c. longitudinal
    d. oblique

15. The endometrium of the uterus is thinnest
    a. just before ovulation.
    b. between ovulation and menstruation.
    c. at the beginning of menstruation.
    d. just after menstruation.

chapter **3**

Prenatal Development

LEARNING ACTIVITIES

1. Match the terms in the left column with their definitions on the right (a–g).

_____ diploid

_____ gamete

_____ haploid

_____ meiosis

_____ mitosis

_____ oogenesis

_____ spermatogenesis

a. normal number of chromosomes in each reproductive cell (23)

b. normal number of chromosomes in each somatic cell (46)

c. cell division in sex cells (gametes)

d. cell division in ordinary body (somatic) cells

e. formation of spermatozoa

f. formation of ova

g. an ovum or spermatozoan

2. a. Spermatogenesis results in the formation of how many spermatids? __________

   b. Each spermatid contains __________ autosomes and either a(n) __________ or a(n) __________ sex chromosome.

3. a. Oogenesis results in the formation of how many ova? __________ How many polar bodies? __________

   b. Each ovum contains __________ autosomes and an __________ sex chromosome.

4. a. An ovum survives about __________ hours after ovulation.

   b. Sperm survive up to __________ hours after ejaculation.

Student Name Shirley Williams SPN.

5. a. If the ovum is fertilized by a sperm bearing a Y chromosome, the baby will be a male.

   b. If the ovum is fertilized by a sperm bearing an X chromosome, the baby will be a female.

   c. What influence, if any, does the woman have on the sex of the baby that is conceived?

   The mother has some influence on which sperm fertilizes the mature ovum.

6. Fertilization usually occurs in the fallopian tube. The fertilized ovum usually implants in the upper section of the posterior uterus.

7. Match the terms in the left column with their definitions on the right (a–i).

A	amnion	a.	inner fetal membrane
____	blastocyst	b.	outer fetal membrane
D	blastomere	c.	solid cluster of cells
B	chorion	d.	eight-cell stage of prenatal development
____	decidua	e.	finger-like projections on the outer part of the placenta
F	embryo	f.	prenatal development from three weeks until the end of the eighth week after fertilization
G	fetus	g.	prenatal development from the ninth week after fertilization until birth
C	morula	h.	uterine lining after implantation
E	villi	i.	zygote containing an inner cell mass that will develop into the embryo

+4 41

8. The normal amount of amniotic fluid near the end of pregnancy is about 00 ml.

9. List the five functions of amniotic fluid.

   a. Maintain an even temperature
   b. Prevent the amniotic sac from adhering to the fetal skin
   c. allow symmetrical growth
   d. Allow buoyancy and fetal movement
   e. act as a cushion to protect the fetus from injury

10. Red blood cells are formed by the ________________________ for the first six weeks after gestation and then are formed by the ________________________ until the 12th week. After 12 weeks, red blood cell production occurs in the ____________.

11. List the tissues that form from each of the three primary germ layers.

Ectoderm

pg. 42

a. Outer layer of skin
b. Oil glands + hair follicles of skin
c. Nails + hair
d. External sense organs
e. Mucous membrane of mouth + anus

Mesoderm

a. True skin
b. Skeleton
c. Bone + cartilage
d. Connective tissue
e. Muscles
f. Blood + blood vessels
g. Kidneys + gonads

Endoderm

a. Lining of trachea, pharynx, + bronchi
b. Lining of digestive tract
c. Lining of bladder + urethra

12. List four functions of the placenta.

pg. 42

a. Respiration
b. nutrition
c. excretion
d. Endocrine gland

Student Name Shirley Williams S.P.N.

13. Describe the functions of each of the four following placental hormones during pregnancy.

a. Progesterone Reduce uterine contractions to prevent spontaneous abortion maintain uterine lining for implantation of the zygote. Prepares the glands of the breast for lactation.

b. Estrogens Stimulates uterine growth, increases the blood flow to uterine vessels + stimulates development of the breast ducts to prepare for lactation.

c. Human chorionic gonadotropin (hCG) Causes the corpus luteum to persist + to continue production of estrogen + progesterone.

d. Human placental lactogen (hPL) The hPL stimulates adjustments in the mother's metabolism, making more glucose available to meet fetal energy needs.

14. Label each of the structures listed below on the drawing provided. Color areas to indicate high (red), medium (purple), and low (blue) fetal blood oxygenation.

a.	ductus venosus	e.	placenta
b.	ductus arteriosus	f.	superior vena cava
c.	foramen ovale	g.	umbilical arteries
d.	inferior vena cava	h.	umbilical vein

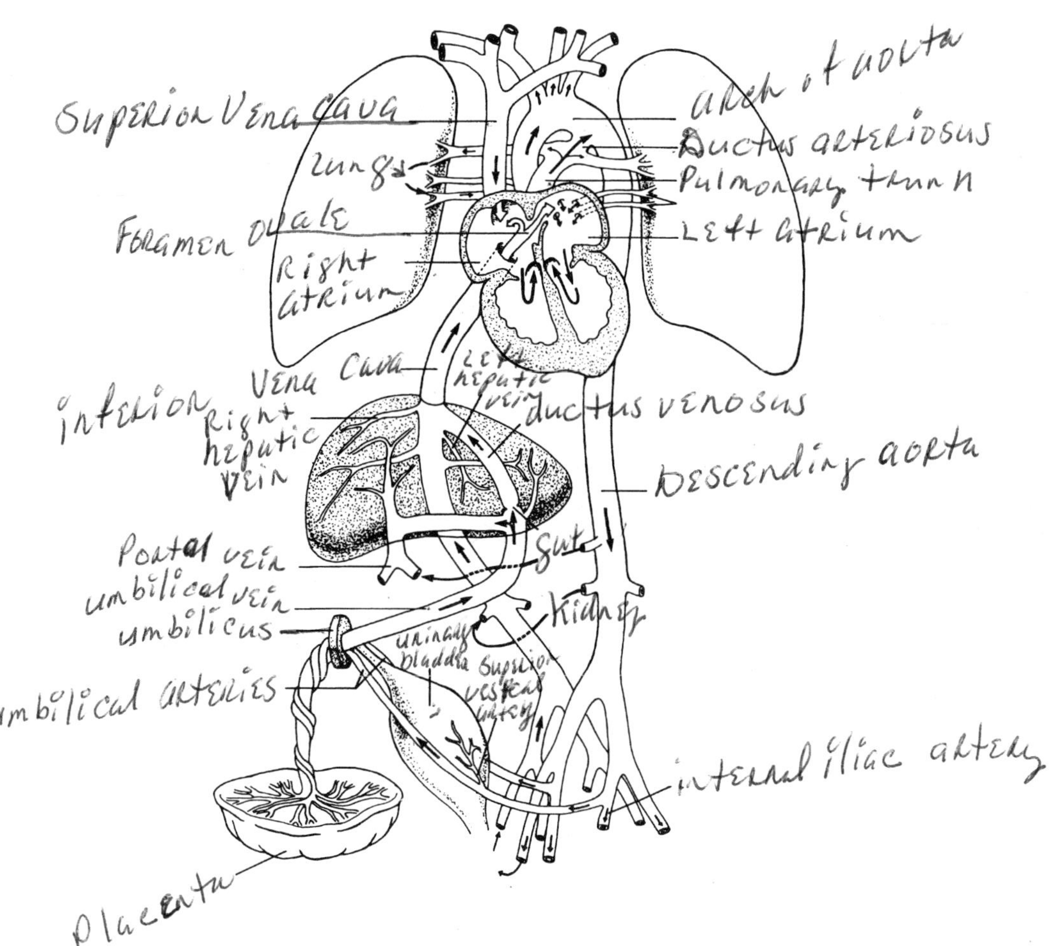

15. The umbilical cord should have ONE vein(s) and TWO artery(ies).

16. State the age when each fetal circulatory structure closes functionally and permanently.

Pg 414

		Functionally	Permanently
a.	ductus arteriosus	diverts blood from pulmonary artery into aorta	
b.	ductus venosus	diverts blood away from the liver as it returns to the placenta	
c.	foramen ovale	divert blood from (R) atrium to the (L) atrium	

17. Match the prenatal ages (fertilization age) with their development characteristics on the right (a–h).

H 3 weeks
A 6 weeks
E 8 weeks
F 10 weeks
G 16 weeks
B 20 weeks
C 28 weeks
D 38 weeks

a. fetal circulation fully established
b. midpoint of pregnancy
c. testes descend into scrotum
d. firm ears, many sole creases
e. tubular heart begins beating; earliest evidence of brain and spinal cord
f. intestines enclosed within abdomen
g. fetal sex can be determined by examining external genitalia
h. heart has all four chambers

18. Match the placental or fetal structures and substances with their descriptions on the right (a–f).

A brown fat
F meconium
E surfactant
C placental membrane
D vernix
B Wharton's jelly

a. heat-producing substance that prevents newborn cold stress
b. substance that protects umbilical vessels between the placenta and fetus
c. structure that keeps maternal and fetal blood separate
d. protective cheese-like fetal skin coating
e. phospholipids that coat the interior of the lung alveoli
f. fetal intestinal contents

Student Name Shirley Williams S.P.N.

19. Describe the differences between monozygotic (identical) and dizygotic (fraternal) twins in terms of the following characteristics.

pg 49-50

	Characteristic	**Monozygotic**	**Dizygotic**
a.	Same sex or different	Two fetuses that develop from a single divided fertilized ovum	fetuses that develop from two fertilized ova
b.	Number of fertilized ova	single ova	two ova
c.	Number of placentas	one	two
d.	Number of membranes	one	two
e.	Number of umbilical cords	one	two

THINKING CRITICALLY

1. A woman comes to the family planning clinic where you work. She wants to try a natural method of birth control rather than use artificial methods of contraception. What facts must you know about the survival time of the ovum and sperm to help your client effectively use this form of family planning? See text, Chapter 11, if you would like further information about natural family planning.

2. Your friend is disappointed because she has just had her fourth girl. "My husband wants a son so much," she says. "I feel terrible that I can't have a boy for him." How would you respond to your friend?

OTHER LEARNING ACTIVITY

1. Examine a placenta, particularly the insertion of the umbilical cord into the placenta. Identify the following structures.

   a. amniotic membranes – amniotic sac (bag of water)

   b. fetal side – chorionic villi + the chorionic blood vessels.

   c. maternal side – arises from the decidua basalis + has a beefy red appearance.

   d. umbilical vein – one vein returns blood to the fetus

   e. umbilical arteries – two carry blood away from the fetus

   f. Wharton's jelly – covers + cushions the cord vessels + keeps the three vessels separated.

REVIEW QUESTIONS

1. Between the third and the eighth week of pregnancy, the developing baby is known as

   a a gamete.

   b. a zygote.

   c. an embryo.

   d. a fetus.

2. Cell division that results in the formation of gametes is known as

   a. mitosis.

   b. meiosis.

   c. diplosis.

   d. haplosis.

3. Normal human sperm and ova should each contain ________ chromosomes.

   a. 23

   b. 46

   c. 69

   d. 92

4. Which sex chromosome combination results in conception of a male?

   a. XX

   b. XY

   c. YY

   d. XO

5. Hereditary or genetic traits are passed from one generation to the next within the

   a. chromosomes.

   b. zygote.

   c. chorionic villi.

   d. somatic cells.

6. After six weeks gestation, fetal red blood cells are manufactured in the

   a. placenta.

   b. liver.

   c. heart.

   d. blastocyst.

7. The purpose of the polar bodies is to

   a. produce estrogen and progesterone.

   b. nourish the zygote before implantation.

   c. eliminate excess female chromosomes.

   d. promote implantation in the best location.

8. The outer fetal membrane is the

   a. amnion.

   b. chorion.

   c. syncytium.

   d. vernix.

9. The primary function of Wharton's jelly is to

   a. keep the umbilical vessels from being compressed.

   b. prevent the fetal membranes from adhering to the fetal skin.

   c. separate maternal blood from fetal blood in the placenta.

   d. carry fetal waste products back to the placenta.

10. Most fetal blood bypasses the lungs by way of the

    a. ductus venosus.

    b. ductus arteriosus.

    c. umbilical vein.

    d. umbilical artery.

Student Name Shirley Williams S.P.N.

11. The fetal circulatory structure that carries blood with the lowest oxygen saturation is the
    a. umbilical vein.
    b. umbilical artery.
    c. ductus venosus.
    d. ductus arteriosus.

12. After fertilization, the zygote grows by
    a. meiosis.
    b. mitosis.
    c. oogenesis.
    d. gametogenesis.

13. The foramen ovale closes permanently in about ________ after birth.
    a. one hour
    b. one day
    c. three weeks
    d. three months

14. The primary purpose of amniotic fluid is to
    a. speed maturation of fetal lungs.
    b. prevent cold stress after birth.
    c. protect the fetus during development.
    d. produce hormones to maintain pregnancy.

15. Fetal waste products are disposed of by the
    a. fetal liver.
    b. placenta.
    c. yolk sac.
    d. endoderm.

16. Inadequate progesterone is likely to result in
    a. release of multiple ova.
    b. spontaneous abortion.
    c. persistence of the corpus luteum.
    d. a mixture of maternal and fetal blood.

17. Fraternal (dizygotic) twins result when
    a. one sperm fertilizes one ovum.
    b. two sperm fertilize one ovum.
    c. one sperm fertilizes two ova
    d. two sperm fertilize two ova.

18. The sex of identical (monozygotic) twins
    a. is always the same.
    b. may or may not be the same.
    c. is always different.

19. An infant born at 30 weeks gestation is likely to have respiratory distress because
    a. excess brown fat limits diaphragm movement.
    b. inadequate surfactant reduces lung expansion.
    c. the placenta does not pass enough meconium to the lungs.
    d. excess vernix enters the airways during birth.

20. Contents of the fetal intestinal tract are known as
    a. meconium.
    b. lanugo.
    c. vernix.
    d. endoderm.

chapter **4**

Prenatal Care and Adaptations to Pregnancy

LEARNING ACTIVITIES

1. Match the terms in the left column with their definitions on the right (a–g).

A colostrum
C hemorrhoids
G mucous plug
D pseudoanemia
E pica
B spider nevi
F trimester

a. breast secretion that precedes milk; rich in antibodies
b. red elevations of skin with lines radiating from center
c. varicose veins of rectum and anus
d. anemia occurring because red cells increase less than plasma volume
e. ingestion of nonfood substances
f. 13-week period of pregnancy
g. seals cervical canal during pregnancy

2. Match the terms describing a woman's obstetrical history with their definitions on the right (a–g).

A gravida
C multigravida
G multipara
D nullipara
E para
B primigravida
F primipara

a. pregnant woman
b. woman pregnant for the first time
c. woman pregnant for the second or subsequent time
d. woman who has not delivered a pregnancy of at least 20 weeks gestation
e. woman who delivered one or more pregnancies after at least 20 weeks gestation
f. woman who has delivered one pregnancy of at least 20 weeks gestation
g. woman who has delivered two or more pregnancies of at least 20 weeks gestation

Student Name Shirley Williams S.P.N.

3. Nagele's Rule is a formula used to calculate a woman's estimated date of delivery (EDD). Describe how to use this formula.

Determine first day of the last normal menstrual period (LNMP), count backward 3 months, add 7 days, correct the year if needed.

4. Describe the presumptive signs of pregnancy.

a. amenorrhea
b. nausea
c. Breast changes
d. Pigmentation changes
e. urgency of urination
f. Fatigue
g. drowsiness

These signs are called *presumptive* because these are common during pregnancy but often can have other causes as well.

5. Describe the probable signs of pregnancy.

a. Goodell's sign (softening of the cervix)
b. Chadwick's sign (purplish or bluish discoloration of the cervix)
c. Hegar's sign (softening of the ↓ uterine segment)
d. abdominal & uterine enlargement
e. Braxton Hicks (uterine contractions that begin 2nd trimester)
f. Ballottement (light tap on the cervix & rebounds quickly)
g. Fetal outline (palpation after the 24th wk.)
h. abdominal striae (stretch marks)
i. Pregnancy test.
j. McDonald sign

These signs are called *probable* because they indication of pregnancy provide stronger evidence of pregnancy.

6. Describe positive signs of pregnancy. At what time during pregnancy can each be detected?

   a. Fetal heartbeat (may be detected as early as 10 weeks of pregnancy by using a Doppler device.

   b. Fetal movement (can be felt by a trained examiner in the 2nd trimester.

   c. Identification of the embryo or fetus (ultrasound observation + photography of the gestational sac is possible as early as 4-5 weeks of gestation.

7. Match the signs and symptoms of pregnancy with their descriptions on the right (a–l).

   B abdominal striae
   H amenorrhea
   C ballottement
   E Braxton-Hicks contractions
   A Chadwick's sign
   L chloasma gravidarum
   G funic souffle
   I Goodell's sign
   D Hegar's sign
   J linea nigra
   K quickening
   F uterine souffle

   a. bluish color of cervix, vagina, and vulva
   b. stretch marks
   c. rebound of fetal part when tapped by examining finger during vaginal examination
   d. softened lower uterus
   e. irregular painless uterine contractions
   f. blowing sound heard over uterus
   g. swishing sound of blood circulating through umbilical cord
   h. cessation of menses
   i. softened cervix and vagina
   j. darker pigmented line in midline of abdomen
   k. movement of fetus felt by mother
   l. brownish pigmentation of face ("mask of pregnancy")

8. a. Oxytocin is the hormone detected in a positive pregnancy test.

   b. Two body fluids used for pregnancy tests are Blood and Urine.

9. Describe changes that occur in the reproductive organs during pregnancy.

   a. Uterus

   Size: Increases in size

   Weight: 1000g (2.2 pounds)

   Capacity: 5000 mL (5 quarts)

Student Name Shirley Williams S.P.N.

b. Cervix change in color + consistency

c. Ovaries do not produce ova (eggs) during pregnancy

d. Vagina blood supply ↑ causing bluish color of Chadwick's sign.

10. Describe changes in other body systems during pregnancy.

a. Breasts ↑ levels of estrogen + progesterone prepare the breasts for lactation.

b. Respiratory Pregnant woman respiratory rate ↑ slightly Dyspnea may occur until the fetus descends into the pelvis, relieving upward pressure on the diaphragm.

c. Cardiovascular Cardiac output ↑ because more blood is pumped from the heart c̄ each contraction + the pulse rate ↑ by 10 to 15 beats/min.

d. Gastrointestinal growing uterus displaces the stomach + intestines toward the back + sides of the abdomen. ↑ salivary secretion sometime affect taste + smell.

e. Urinary system excretes waste products for both the mother + fetus during pregnancy. The glomerular filtration rate of the kidney rises.

f. Integumentary and skeletal The ↑ levels of hormones produced during pregnancy cause a variety of temporary changes in the skin. (integument) The woman's posture changes as her baby grows c̄ in the uterus.

11. Describe the recommended weight gain if the woman's prepregnancy weight is as follows:

a. normal: 25 to 35 pounds

b. underweight: 28 to 40 pounds

c. overweight: 15 to 25 pounds

12. The recommended calorie increase during pregnancy is 300 calories per day.

13. For the following four nutrients, state the amount needed during pregnancy for an adult and list key food sources for each nutrient.

   a. Protein

   Amount: An intake of 60 g/day

   Sources: meat, fish, poultry + dairy products, beans, lentils + other legumes; breads + cereals; + seeds + nuts, combined c̄ another plant or animal protein

   b. Calcium

   Amount: An intake of 1200 mg

   Sources: Dairy products, enriched cereals, legumes, nuts, dried fruits, broccoli, green leafy vegetables + canned salmon + sardines that contains bones.

   c. Iron

   Amount: Recommended allowance is 30 mg/day

   Sources: Iron supplement is prescribe, 30 mg/day beginning in the 2nd trimester, after morning sickness.

   d. Folic acid

   Amount: RDA for a pregnant woman 400 µg (0.4 mg)

   Sources: liver, kidney + lima beans, fresh, dark-green leafy vegetables; lean beef; potatoes; whole-wheat bread; dried beans + peanuts.

14. List at least three measures the nurse can teach a woman to relieve each common pregnancy discomfort. Note any related abnormal signs or symptoms that should be reported.

   a. Nausea

   Eat dry toast or cracker before getting out of bed.
   Drink fluids between meals instead of c̄ meals.
   Eat small, frequent meals.
   Avoid fried, greasy or spicy food.
   Vomiting that significantly interferes c̄ food + fluid intake is not normal + should be be reported.

Student Name Shirley Williams S.P.N.

b. Increased vaginal discharge

(1) Bathe or shower daily, (2) Wear loose-fitting cotton panties, (3) Wipe perineal area from front to back after toileting. yellow discharge c̄ foul odor, accompanied by itching + inflammation suggests vaginal infection + should be reported.

c. Fatigue

(1) Try to get at least 8 to 10 hrs of sleep @ night.
(2) Take nap during the day if possible.
(3) Use measures such as relaxation techniques, meditation or change of scenery.

d. Backache

Squat rather than bend over when picking up objects. When sitting, support the arms, feet, + back c̄ pillows as needed

e. Constipation Drink 6-8 glasses of H_2O daily, include roughage, moderate exercise, sit on toilet c̄ feet on stool, maintain regular position, use relaxation tech./deep breathing, don't take stool softeners or meds s̄ doc. permission

f. Varicose veins aching legs c̄ tenderness, avoid obesity, lengthy standing or sitting, constrictive clothing, avoid bearing down c̄ bowel movements. Moderate exercise, rest c̄ legs elevated, support stocking

g. Heartburn avoid gas-forming or fatty foods, lg. meals, good posture. Tx: Take only antiacids prescribed by physician, baking soda + alkaseltzers are contraindicated, drink hot tea, or chew gum.

h. Dyspnea

avoid anemia, Tx: Refer to physician if symptoms persist, practice good posture, sleep c̄ extra pillows, avoid overloading the stomach, stop or ↓ smoking.

i. Leg cramps Teach to avoid pointing the toes when stretching the legs. When walking lead c̄ heel first, avoid fatigue + cold legs, diet adequate in calcium.

j. Edema of the legs good posture, avoid prolonged standing or sitting, moderate exercise, avoid constrictive clothing, maintain fluid intake, elt pt. [illegible] generalized edema notify physician. Put on support stocking before getting up, lay down + prop feet against the wall.

15. Describe the common emotional reactions of a woman during each trimester of pregnancy.

a. First The woman may have difficulty believing that she's pregnant during early pregnancy, because she may not feel much different.

b. Second They have resolved many of their earlier feeling of ambivalence. They take on the role of a expected mother wholeheartedly.

c. Third The mother begins to separate herself from the pregnancy + commit herself to the care of an infant. She + her partner begin making concrete preparatio for the baby's arrival.

THINKING CRITICALLY

1. Today is June 19. A woman is admitted to the hospital in labor. She tells you that her "due date" is June 26. How many weeks pregnant is the woman? 38 wks.

2. If a woman's expected date of delivery is July 21, what was the first day of her last menstrual period? May 28,

3. Have a discussion group that contains both men and women who have had children (they do not have to be nurses or nursing students). Discuss the parts fathers played in any births. Explore the feelings of men in the group about how they view their role in childbirth.

Student Name Shirley Williams S.P.N.

CASE STUDIES

1. Rosa Garza comes to the clinic for a regular visit at 26 weeks gestation. Her weight gain has been normal (17 pounds), but Rosa tells you that her mother cautioned her not to gain more than 20 pounds or it will be hard to lose the weight after she gives birth. "My mother said that I should not eat salt and that the doctor will probably give me 'water pills' if I gain too much weight." What teaching should you give Rosa about each of her concerns? ~~Obes~~: overweight women should gain 15-25 lbs.

    a. weight gain - women of normal wt. should gain 25-35 lbs. women underweight should gain 28-40 lbs.

    b. salt (sodium) intake is essential for maintaining normal sodium levels in plasma, bone, brain + muscle.

    c. diuretics ("water pills") are not recommended for the healthy pregnant woman, because they reduce fluids necessary for the fetus.

2. Lauren Holt, 30 years old, is pregnant for the first time. She describes herself as a vegetarian, although she says she occasionally eats dairy products and eggs. What nutritional advice can the nurse provide, considering Lauren's pregnancy needs and her food preferences? Teach her about non-meat protein, to ensure that her protein needs are met.

OTHER LEARNING ACTIVITIES

1. Each date below represents the first day of a woman's last menstrual period. Use a wheel to calculate the expected date of delivery for each. If you have access to an electronic gestation calculator, use it to make the same calculations. Using today's date, figure how many weeks the pregnancy has advanced.

    a. January 18

    b. July 13

    c. December 30

2. Use the TPAL system to describe each of the following pregnancy histories.

    a. A woman is pregnant for the fourth time. She had one spontaneous abortion, one child born at 32 weeks gestation who is living, and another living child born at 41 weeks gestation.

    b. A woman is 32 weeks pregnant with her second pregnancy. Her first pregnancy ended with a spontaneous abortion at 8 weeks gestation.

REVIEW QUESTIONS

1. When a woman is 20 weeks pregnant, she is expected to experience
   - a. nausea and vomiting.
   - b. movement of the fetus.
   - c. burning during urination.
   - d. heavy vaginal discharge.
2. A woman is 12 weeks pregnant. During a prenatal visit, she tells the nurse she is worried that her baby might not be normal. How should the nurse interpret this statement?
   - a. Concerns about fetal well-being and normality are common during early pregnancy.
   - b. It is unusual for women to have these feelings because they do not perceive the baby as "real."
   - c. She may have underlying rejection of the fetus that is being expressed in this way.
   - d. Her image of the fetus is expected to be more realistic at this time.
3. A woman's emotional reaction during the second trimester of pregnancy is characterized by
   - a. fear for her safety during labor.
   - b. passive and dependent behavior.
   - c. feelings of being unattractive.
   - d. dramatic changes in her moods.
4. The purpose of the mucous plug is to
   - a. increase the blood supply to the uterus.
   - b. block infection of the uterus.
   - c. soften and stretch the cervix.
   - d. lubricate the vaginal walls.
5. While lying on the examining table during her prenatal check, a woman complains of being dizzy and weak. She is pale and her skin is moist. The best nursing intervention to relieve her symptoms is to
   - a. have her turn to her side.
   - b. tell her to take deep breaths.
   - c. help her sit up on the table.
   - d. elevate her feet and legs.
6. A woman who is underweight at the beginning of pregnancy should gain how much weight during pregnancy?
   - a. 15–25 pounds
   - b. 25–35 pounds
   - c. 28–40 pounds
   - d. more than 40 pounds
7. To ensure that a woman has adequate iron intake during pregnancy, it is often recommended that she
   - a. drink at least one quart of milk per day.
   - b. take 30 mg of an iron supplement daily.
   - c. eat combinations of meat and grains.
   - d. eat 18 mg of iron daily in a variety of foods.
8. What should the nurse teach a pregnant woman about caring for varicose veins in her legs?
   - a. Apply warm packs to the legs.
   - b. Sit down as much as possible.
   - c. Stretch the legs while pointing toes.
   - d. Elevate the legs when sitting.
9. The primary goal of prenatal care is to assure the woman of
   - a. labor with a minimum of pain.
   - b. the healthiest outcome possible.
   - c. improved long-term nutrition.
   - d. minimal pregnancy discomforts.

Student Name Shirley Williams S.P.N

10. A woman who is pregnant with her first baby is called a
    a. multigravida.
    b. para.
    c. nullipara.
    d. primipara.

11. Which of these foods are the highest in iron?
    a. Citrus fruits and melons
    b. Milk, cheese, and other dairy products
    c. Grains and deep yellow vegetables
    d. Meat and dark green vegetables

12. Adequate stores of folic acid are needed before conception to
    a. promote adequate expansion of the blood volume.
    b. reduce nausea and vomiting in the first trimester.
    c. limit depletion of calcium from the mother's teeth.
    d. reduce the risk for fetal neural tube defects.

13. The best goal for the nursing diagnosis Nutrition: Less than Body Requirements, Altered, related to low prepregnancy weight, is that the client will
    a. identify recommended nutrient intake during pregnancy.
    b. gain at least 28 pounds by the end of pregnancy.
    c. recognize that good nutrition promotes maternal and fetal health.
    d. state the appropriate calorie increase for pregnancy.

14. The first day of a woman's last menstrual period was September 5. Her estimated date of delivery (EDD) is
    a April 12.
    b. May 5.
    c. June 12.
    d. July 16.

15. Choose the most appropriate teaching for the nursing diagnosis of Constipation, related to effects of pregnancy.
    a. Take a mild laxative no more than three times per week.
    b. Eat several servings of raw fruits and vegetables each day.
    c. Limit fluids to one quart each day, taken between meals.
    d. Wait until the environment is quiet before defecating.

16. The expectant mother is more likely to have leg cramps if she
    a. does not take her iron supplement each day.
    b. increases her fluid intake to eight glasses per day.
    c. elevates her legs without a sharp bend at the knee.
    d. drinks more than one quart of milk each day.

17. A pregnant woman calls the prenatal clinic and says she has a profuse yellow vaginal discharge. The nurse should instruct the woman to
    a. douche with a commercial vinegar and water solution.
    b. avoid sexual intercourse until the symptoms go away.
    c. wear cotton panties that allow adequate air circulation.
    d. come to the clinic for further evaluation by the physician.

18. The most appropriate teaching for relief of nausea during early pregnancy is to

    a. divide daily food intake into several small meals.

    b. sit upright for 30–60 minutes after meals.

    c. drink at least eight ounces of liquid with each meal.

    d. eat dry toast or crackers each night before sleep.

19. A pregnant woman is concerned about the "ugly brown spots" on her face. The nurse should teach her that

    a. unscented skin lotions may reduce the darkness of the areas.

    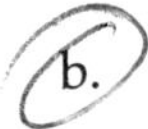

    b. these are temporary changes due to increased hormones.

    c. she should avoid wearing makeup until the areas fade.

    d. iron supplements sometimes cause temporary skin darkening.

20. It is important to maintain adequate fluid intake during pregnancy primarily to prevent

    a. orthostatic hypotension.

    b. edema of the feet and legs.

    c. nausea and vomiting.

    d. urinary tract infection.

Student Name Shirley Williams S.P.N.

chapter **5**

Nursing Care of Women with Complications During Pregnancy

LEARNING ACTIVITIES

1. Match the terms in the left column with their definitions on the right (a–f).

B abruptio placentae
F ectopic pregnancy
E hyperemesis gravidarum
D incompetent cervix
A placenta previa
C spontaneous abortion

a. placental attachment in the lower uterus
b. premature separation of the placenta that is normally attached
c. "miscarriage," or a pregnancy that unintentionally ends before 20 weeks
d. failure of the cervix to remain closed until the fetus reaches term
e. excessive nausea and vomiting during pregnancy
f. development of the fetus outside the uterus

2. List four appropriate nursing interventions for the woman with hyperemesis gravidarum.

a. Eat dry toast or crackers before getting out of bed in the morning.

b. Drink fluids between meals instead of c̄ meals.

c. Eat small frequent meals.

d. Avoid fried, greasy, or spicy foods + foods c̄ strong odors, such as cabbage + onions.

3. Match the types of spontaneous abortion with their descriptions on the right (a–f).

B threatened
F incomplete
D inevitable
C complete
E missed
A recurrent

a. three or more consecutive spontaneous abortions
b. vaginal bleeding without dilation of the cervix or passage of tissue
c. passage of all products of conception
d. bleeding and cramping with cervical dilation but no passage of tissue
e. retention of the dead fetus in the uterus
f. bleeding and cramping with passage of some tissue

4. Describe important teaching for a woman after spontaneous abortion for each aspect listed.

a. Bleeding Report ↑ bleeding, Do not use tampons, which cause infection.

b. Temperature Take q 8 hours for 3 days, Report signs of infection (temp. 100.4 or ↑, foul odor or brownish color of vaginal drainage.

c. Resuming sexual activity as recommended by the physician, (usually after the bleeding has ~~stop~~ stopped.)

d. Contraception Return to physician for f/up & contraception information.

5. An ectopic pregnancy usually occurs in the fallopian tube (tubal pregnancy).

6. The primary nursing observation related to ectopic pregnancy is for ________________.

7. Describe each characteristic of gestational trophoblastic disease.

a. Uterine size Larger than expected for gestation

b. Ultrasound appearance snowstorm pattern on ultrasound c̄ no developing baby in the uterus

c. Human chorionic gonadotropin (hCG) levels Higher than expected

d. Presence of vomiting ________________

RH immune globin is prescribed for RH-negative woman.

Student Name Shing Williams S.P.N.

e. Blood pressure

f. Risk for cancer

8. Describe the location of each type of placenta previa.

a. Marginal Placenta reaches the edge of the cervical opening

b. Partial Placenta partly covers the cervical opening

c. Total Placenta completely covers the cervical opening

9. How does placenta previa differ from abruptio placentae in each of the following characteristics?

a. Pain It is a painless vaginal bleeding + Abruptio Placenta has abdominal or low back pain.

b. Consistency of the uterus Abruptio Placenta the uterus is tender + is tie (boardlike)

c. Blood coagulation

10. List six or more factors that increase a woman's risk for development of pregnancy-induced hypertension (PIH).

a. First pregnancy

b. African American

c. Family history of PIH

d. Age over 40 years

e. Multifetal pregnancy (twins)

f. Diabetes Mellitus

11. Describe each variation of pregnancy-induced hypertension.

    a. Preeclampsia Renal involvement leads to proteinuria

    b. Eclampsia Occurs when the woman has one or more generalized tonic-clonic seizures.

    c. HELLP involves hemolysis (breakage of erythrocytes), elevated liver enzymes + low platelets

12. What blood pressure elevation is significant during pregnancy?

    ____

13. Differentiate between mild and severe preeclampsia for the following characteristics.

    a. Blood pressure Systolic BP 160mm Hg < / Severe > 160mm Hg Diastolic < 100mm Hg / Severe > 110mm Hg

    b. Edema (Severe) "pitting" / (mild) Sudden excessive wt. gain is first sign of fluid retention

    c. Proteinuria (mild) Trace / Severe > 5g/24h

    ____

14. Describe other manifestations of severe preeclampsia.

    a. Central nervous system changes Deep tendon reflexes become hyperactive because of CNS irritability.

    b. Visual disturbances blurred or double vision or "spots before the eyes" occur because of arterial spasm + edema of the retina.

    c. Urine output ↓ blood flow to the kidney reduces urine production + worsens hypertension.

    d. Abdominal pain Epigastric pain or nausea occur because of liver edema, ischemia + necrosis + often precede convulsion

15. What is the significance of abdominal pain or visual disturbances in a woman with preeclampsia? ______________________________

    ____

Student Name Shirley Williams S.P.N

16. What is the benefit of activity restriction in treatment of preeclampsia?

Activity restriction allows blood that would be circulated to skeletal muscles to be conserved for circulation to the mother's vital organs & the placenta.

17. a. What is the purpose of magnesium sulfate in the treatment of PIH?

Magnesium sulfate is an anticonvulsant given to prevent seizures.

b. What drug should be on hand if a woman is receiving magnesium sulfate?

Calcium Gluconate + Oxytocin

18. Explain the frequency and purpose of the following nursing assessments for a woman who is receiving magnesium sulfate.

a. Vital signs (v) q 4hrs, Rising hypertension, particularly if blood pressure is 160/100 or higher, signs of magnesium ~~sulfate~~ toxicity.

b. Deep tendon reflexes (v) q 1 to 4 hrs Signs of CNS irritability, such as facial twitching or hyperactive D.T.R.

c. Urine output and protein content Urine output q h, protein in urine after each void. / decreased urine output, especially if less than 25mL/hr.

19. a. Rh blood incompatibility can only occur if the mother is Rh − negative and the fetus is Rh − positive.

b. The drug given to prevent Rh incompatibility is Rh immune globulin (RhoGAM).

c. List four instances in which the drug listed in part (b) is indicated.

Birth

Abortion (spontaneous or induced)

Episodes of bleeding

Amniocentesis

20. a. ABO incompatibility is more likely to occur in which maternal blood group or groups? group O blood (mother) (fetus) has group A, B or AB blood

    b. In which fetal blood group or groups? group A, B or AB groups

21. Which type of diabetes mellitus is most common during pregnancy?

    Gestational diabetes Mellitus (GDM)

22. a. Why is glucose monitored by blood testing during pregnancy?

    ____

    ____

    b. Does urine testing have a place in diabetes management during pregnancy?

    ____

23. The only drug used to lower the blood glucose during pregnancy is insulin because it dose not cross the placenta.

24. List three cardiac conditions that may complicate pregnancy.

    a. Rheumatic fever

    b. Congential heart defects

    c. Mitral valve prolapse

25. How may normal changes of pregnancy affect the woman with heart disease?

    ____

    ____

    ____

26. Why is a woman with heart disease predisposed to congestive heart failure after birth?

    Excess interstitial fluid rapidly returns to the circulation after birth, predisposing the woman to circulatory overload during postpartum period.

27. Describe the use of the following drugs for the pregnant woman who has heart disease.

    a. Heparin To prevent clot formation

    b. Antibiotics Give during intrapartum period to prevent infection.

    c. Diuretics for fluid overload.

Student Name [Shirley Williams S.N.]

28. List three reasons why a pregnant woman needs increased iron.

    a. [for RBC own increase blood volume]

    b. [for transfer to the fetus]

    c. [for a cushion against the blood loss @ birth.]

29. A hemoglobin level lower than [10.5 to 11] g/dl indicates anemia during pregnancy.

30. List foods high in the following nutrients.

    a. Iron [Meat, chicken, fish, liver, legumes, green leafy vegetables, whole or enriched grain products, nuts, blackstrap molasses, tofu, eggs, dried fruits + food cooked in cast iron.]

    b. Vitamin C [citrus fruits + juices, strawberries, cantaloupe, cabbage, green + red peppers, tomatoes, potatoes, green leafy vegetables]

    c. Folic acid [green leafy vegetables, asparagus, green beans, fruits, whole grains, liver, legumes, yeast.]

31. An iron supplement should not be taken with milk because [it will not absorbed easily.].

32. Match each infection with the method to prevent infection of the fetus or newborn on the right (a–d).

    [C] toxoplasmosis

    [B] rubella

    [D] cytomegalovirus

    [A] herpes

    a. deliver infant by cesarean birth if the woman has genital lesions when labor begins

    b. immunize children; immunize nonimmune woman after birth

    c. wash hands and surfaces after handling raw meat; cook meat thoroughly; avoid cat litter

    d. no effective prevention or treatment

33. What are the recommendations to prevent hepatitis-B in the newborn?

Routine immunization c̄ hepatitis B vaccine for all newborns @ birth, 1 to 2 months & 6 to 18 months

34. Why does it require several months to determine if an infant born to an HIV-positive mother is infected?

35. What teaching about the following is appropriate to prevent the spread of AIDS?

a. Drug abuse avoid ~~sharing~~ sharing needles

b. Sexual intercourse use a latex condom, avoid oral sex.

36. The infant born to a woman with group B *Streptococcus* infection is at risk for ______.

37. For each of the following sexually transmitted diseases (STDs), describe (a) the effects on the mother, (b) the effects on the fetus or newborn, and (c) the treatment.

Syphilis

a. a generalized rash, on palms & soles as well as on the body, 4-6 wk. later, low fever c̄ rash untreated pt. syphilis may attack the heart & CNS.

b. Transmitted transplacentally, may produce spontaneous abortion preterm labor, stillbirth & congenital syphilis, exposure during 3rd trimester produces enlarge liver, spleen, rash & jaundice

c. Screening during prenatal care is standard treatment with penicillin before 16 wk can prevent fetal infection because the antibiotic crosses the placenta.

Student Name Shirley Williams S.B.N.

Gonorrhea (Cause by the bacterium Neisseria gonorrhoeae)

a. Itching of the vulva, painful urination, may be asymptomatic may cause infertility by blocking the fallopian tubes.

b. Transmitted to the infant during birth by direct contact c̄ the mother's infected birth canal, resulting in eye infection that can cause blindness, may also cause premature rupture of the membrane

c. Treat c̄ ceftriaxone, spectinomycin, or aqueous procaine penicillin (intramuscular) cefixime and ampicillin may be given orally.

Chlamydia (Caused by bacterium Chlamydia trachomatis)

a. Red yellow vaginal discharge, painful frequent urination, or may be asymptomatic, may cause infertility by blocking the ~~fallopian~~ fallopian tubes

b. Transmitted to infant's eyes during birth by contact c̄ mother's infected birth canal, resulting in conjunctivitis, may also result infant pneumonitis, associated c̄ preterm labor, premature rupture membr

c. Treat during pregnancy c̄ erythromycin, tetracycline is effective but should not be taken during pregnancy, eye prophylactic antibiotic ointment is used.

Trichomoniasis (Caused by the protozoon Trichomonas vaginalis)

a. Frothy, gray-green, foul vaginal discharge; perineal itching; reddened skin.

b. Does not cross the placenta; neonatal infection is short-lived; associated c̄ premature rupture of the membrances & postpartum maternal infection.

c. Avoid treatment until after the 1st trimester to prevent adverse drug effects on fetus; clotrimazole (Glyne-Lotrimin) can be given 1st trimester & systemic metronidazole (Flagyl) can be given during 2nd trimester & 3rd. women taking metronidazole should avoid alcohol for 48 hrs after she stops taking the drug.

(caused by the virus, human papillomavirus)
Condylomata acuminata (*genital warts*)

a. Genital warts; cauliflower-like growths, accompanied by itching, vulva pain, + vaginal discharge, associated c̄ development of genital cancer

b. Contact via birth canal can cause laryngeal papillomas, resulting in abnormal cry, voice change, hoarseness, or airway obstruction. Symptom may appear 1 month or more after contact

c. Trichloroacetic acid applied topically to the growths cryotherapy, surgical excision, laser or electrocautery

38. An infant born to a mother with candidiasis may develop a mouth condition called Thrush.

Its appearance resembles milk curds.

39. Bacterial vaginosis is usually treated with Metronidazole (Flagyl) during pregnancy. This drug should be given after the 1st trimester.

40. Why is a pregnant woman more likely to have a urinary tract infection? Because pressure on urinary structure keeps the bladder from emptying completely the ureters dilates + lose motility under the relaxing effect of the hormone progesterone, urine that is retained becomes more alkaline and provides a favorable environment for growth of microorganism.

41. List at least three items the nurse can teach a woman about avoiding a urinary tract infection.

a. Front-to-back direction should be used when doing perineal cleaning or applying + removing perineal pads.

b. Adequate fluid intake promotes frequent voiding, @ least 8 glasses of liquid / d.

c. Urination before intercourse reduces irritation; urinating afterward flushes urine from the bladder.

42. a. Describe the manifestations of fetal alcohol syndrome (FAS).

growth retardation; mental retardation; + facial abnormalities, including a flat, thin upper lip border + downslanting eyes.

Student Name Shirley Williams S.P.N.

b. What is the current recommendation about alcohol intake during pregnancy?

Women should abstain from alcohol use from conception.

43. Match the substances with their potential adverse effects if used during pregnancy on the right (a–d).

C cigarette smoking

A cocaine

B heroin

D marijuana

a. Severe vasoconstriction may cause myocardial infarction, seizures, sudden death, and disrupt placental circulation.

b. Abstinence syndrome may develop in woman or infant if drug is stopped suddenly.

c. Infant may be smaller than normal.

d. There are no clearly documented adverse effects.

44. Describe recommendations to prevent adverse fetal effects resulting from maternal ingestion of the following drugs.

a. Anticonvulsants The physician prescribes the anticonvulsant that is least teratogenic to the fetus while still controlling the mother's seizures

b. Anticoagulants Heparin can not cross the placenta to affect the fetus.

c. Acne medications The woman of childbearing age must use reliable birth control during isotretinoin therapy & for a time afterward to allow the drug to leave the body.

45. What is the priority of medical and nursing care if a pregnant woman suffers trauma?

Placing a small pillow under one hip tilts the heavy uterus off the inferior vena cava to improve blood flow throughout the woman's body to the placenta. Assess for uterine contractions or tenderness, which may indicate onset of labor or abruptio placentae.

THINKING CRITICALLY

1. How might anemia affect a woman who has heart disease?

2. You are helping care for a woman receiving intravenous magnesium sulfate. You note that her urine output has decreased, and was 25 ml during the past hour. What is the significance of your observation? What is the appropriate action? Why?

3. When a couple loses a baby because of spontaneous abortion, how do you think their friends and family are likely to react? What emotional support is appropriate if the woman believes that she should not feel sad because she did not really know the baby yet? How can the nurse help the family cope with this crisis?

CASE STUDY

1. a. Amy Adams, 28 years old, is pregnant for the fifth time. She has had two spontaneous abortions, and one stillborn baby who was born after 35 weeks of pregnancy. Amy's only living child, Sam, weighed 10 pounds, 3 ounces when born at 36 weeks gestation. Amy had hypertension in her pregnancy with Sam and with her stillborn baby. She is at the clinic for a routine prenatal check at 12 weeks. Her weight gain is normal, but she began pregnancy about 25 pounds overweight. All other prenatal checks are normal. Identify three or more factors that predispose Amy to complications in this pregnancy. What prenatal assessments may identify these complications early? What danger signals in pregnancy should you teach Amy?

   b. Amy's pregnancy progresses normally until 28 weeks gestation. A glucose tolerance test was abnormal, and Amy must take insulin injections twice a day to control her gestational diabetes. What teaching will Amy need for this new problem?

   c. Amy is 35 weeks pregnant. Her gestational diabetes has been well controlled, although she has needed higher doses of insulin as pregnancy progressed. She has now developed mild preeclampsia, and her physician advises her to remain on bed rest at home. What teaching is important about Amy's therapy for preeclampsia? How can the nurse help Amy and her family cope with the stresses of her high-risk pregnancy?

OTHER LEARNING ACTIVITIES

1. Assist the experienced nurse in assessing each of these reflexes.
   a. patella
   b. biceps
   c. triceps

2. Study your hospital's policies and procedures for nursing care of a woman who has preeclampsia or eclampsia.

3. Observe the nursing care of a woman who is receiving magnesium sulfate for PIH. What is the reason for each nursing intervention specifically related to magnesium sulfate administration? Did the woman have any of the risk factors for PIH listed in Box 5-3 in the textbook?

Student Name Shirley Williams S.P.N.

4. Visit a public health clinic that treats people with tuberculosis in your area. Do they treat pregnant women at the clinic? Is drug resistance a problem in the people treated there?

REVIEW QUESTIONS

1. A pregnant woman who has insulin-dependent diabetes mellitus asks the nurse why she has needed several increases in her insulin dose during pregnancy. The best answer is that
   a. the changes of pregnancy decrease the body's ability to absorb insulin.
   b. the placenta secretes substances that decrease the effectiveness of insulin.
   c. the fetus does not yet secrete insulin and needs more from the mother.
   d. the pancreas secretes less insulin as pregnancy progresses.

2. During a seizure, the priority nursing action for the pregnant woman is to
   a. maintain client safety.
   b. provide supplemental oxygen.
   c. insert something between her teeth.
   d. give an anticonvulsant medication.

3. The purpose of the biophysical profile (BPP) is to
   a. assess the amount of blood incompatibility between the mother and fetus.
   b. determine if the fetal lungs are mature enough to survive extrauterine life.
   c. determine if the placenta is functioning well enough to support fetal life.
   d. identify congenital abnormalities during early pregnancy.

4. If a pregnant woman is not immune to rubella, the expected action is to
   a. limit her contact with other pregnant women.
   b. immunize her during the postpartum period.
   c. inform her that her baby may have defects.
   d. tell her that there is little risk for problems.

5. Select the most appropriate teaching for the woman who is prone to urinary tract infections.
   a. Use a back-to-front direction when wiping the perineal area.
   b. Eat a diet high in fiber and vitamin C.
   c. Drink eight or more glasses of liquid each day.
   d. Avoid using lubricant during sexual intercourse.

6. If a woman has cardiac disease, the main risks to the fetus are related to
   a. poor oxygenation.
   b. prematurity.
   c. maternal infection.
   d. congenital anomalies.

7. The primary risk when a woman has hyperemesis gravidarum is
   a. vitamin and mineral deficiency.
   b. spontaneous abortion.
   c. fluid and electrolyte imbalance.
   d. intrauterine infection.

8. The most common cause of bleeding in early pregnancy is
   a. hydatidiform mole.
   b. ectopic pregnancy.
   c. placenta previa.
   d. spontaneous abortion.

9. The most important nursing assessment for a woman who is hospitalized with a possible ectopic pregnancy is to observe for
   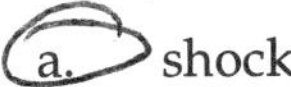
   a. shock.
   b. infection.
   c. dehydration.
   d. acidosis.

10. The nurse should emphasize the importance of long-term follow-up care for the woman who has a hydatidiform mole to detect the occurrence of
   a. recurrent pregnancy.
   b. choriocarcinoma.
   c. hypertension.
   d. continued bleeding.

11. The primary difference between the signs of abruptio placentae and placenta previa is that abruptio placentae involves
   a. bleeding.
   b. infection.
   c. vomiting.
   d. pain.

12. A woman is admitted to the hospital with painless vaginal bleeding in the third trimester of pregnancy. Which test should the nurse expect?
   a. x-ray
   b. ultrasound
   c. vaginal exam
   d. blood count

13. The cause of preeclampsia is
   a. poor nutrition.
   b. excess weight gain.
   c. multiple fetuses.
   d. unknown.

14. A woman who is hospitalized with severe preeclampsia should be closely observed for the onset of
   a. seizures.
   b. proteinuria.
   c. hypotension.
   d. edema.

15. The drug used to reverse magnesium toxicity is
   a. ferrous oxide.
   b. calcium gluconate.
   c. Ringer's lactate.
   d. magnesium chloride.

16. Teaching of the woman who has herpesvirus infection should include
   a. antibiotic treatment of the baby after birth.
   b. the possibility of birth by cesarean delivery.
   c. the minor effects of herpes infection on a newborn.
   d. the minimal type of symptoms in the woman.

17. It is best to treat syphilis during early pregnancy primarily to prevent
   a. infection of the sexual partner.
   b. pelvic inflammatory disease.
   c. eye damage in the newborn.
   d. infection of the fetus.

Student Name Shirley Williams

18. The nurse should expect to teach the pregnant woman with gestational diabetes to monitor her glucose by
    a. assessing blood levels several times a day.
    b. determining levels in the urine twice a day.
    c. having the lab determine fasting glucose levels daily.
    d. keeping a written record of hypoglycemic symptoms.

19. When admitting a woman to the birth unit, the nurse notes on her prenatal record that she has mitral valve prolapse syndrome. The nurse should expect which of the following medical orders for this condition?
    a. prophylactic antibiotic therapy
    b. heparin anticoagulation during labor
    c. restricted intravenous fluid infusion
    d. correction of anemia with blood transfusion

20. Teaching for the pregnant woman who was newly diagnosed with tuberculosis should include
    a. increasing fluid intake to two quarts each day.
    b. the expectation that birth will require a cesarean delivery.
    c. the importance of taking the entire course of medication.
    d. avoiding contact with family members until all medication is taken.

chapter **6**

Nursing Care During Labor and Birth

LEARNING ACTIVITIES

1. List the "4 Ps" of the birth process.
   a. The Powers
   b. The Passage
   c. The Passenger
   d. The Psyche

2. Match the terms in the left column with their definitions on the right (a–f).

F	dilation	a.	length of a labor contraction from beginning to end
A	duration	b.	relaxation period between two labor contractions
C	effacement	c.	thinning of the cervix
E	frequency	d.	strength of labor contractions
D	intensity	e.	time interval from the beginning of one labor contraction until the beginning of the next
B	interval	f.	opening of the cervix

3. The two powers of labor are:
   a. Uterine Contraction
   b. The mother's pushing efforts

4. The amount of cervical effacement is described as a percentage or ~~as~~ or as its estimated length in centimeters.

   The amount of cervical dilation is expressed in centimeters full dilation begin 10cm.

Student Name Shirley Williams SPN.

5. Label each part of the labor contraction cycle on the diagram below.

a. increment
b. acme (peak)
c. decrement
d. frequency
e. duration
f. intensity
g. interval

6. The nurse should promptly report contraction durations longer than ~~q 2 min~~ 90 seconds or intervals shorter than 60 seconds. Why?
Persistent contraction intervals shorter than 60 seconds may reduce fetal oxygen supply.

7. The false pelvis is the upper, flaring part.

The true pelvis is the lower part.

8. Three divisions of the true pelvis are the

a. inlet @ the top
b. The midpelvis (in the middle)
c. Outlet near the perineum.

9. What importance do the sutures and fontanelles of the fetal head have during the birth process?

a. The sutures & fontanels of the fetal head allow it to change shape as it passes through the pelvis (molding).
b. They are important landmarks in determining how the fetus is oriented in the mother's pelvis during birth.

10. Match the terms in the left column with their definitions on the right (a–d).

D attitude
C lie
A position
B presentation

a. orientation of a fixed point on the fetus to the mother's pelvis
b. fetal part first entering the pelvis
c. orientation of the fetus in relation to the mother's spine
d. fetal flexion or extension

11. The abbreviations below describe fetal presentation and position. Spell out each and identify the one describing a breech presentation, the one describing a face presentation, and the one that is the most common of those listed.

a. RSA Right Sacrum Anterior
b. LMT Left Mentum Transverse
c. ROA Right Occiput Anterior
d. LOP Left Occiput Posterior

12. The key difference between true labor and false labor is Change in the Cervix Effacement &/or dilation.

13. Match the mechanisms of labor with their descriptions on the right (a–g).

B descent
E engagement
F flexion
C internal rotation
G extension
A external rotation
D expulsion

a. turning of the fetal head so that it faces one of the mother's thighs
b. downward progress of the fetal presenting part
c. turning of the fetal head within the mother's pelvis
d. birth of the fetal shoulders and body
e. descent of the fetal presenting part to a zero station or lower
f. bending of the fetal head toward the chest
g. pivoting of the fetal neck under the mother's symphysis pubis

14. The first stage of labor lasts from the onset [illegible] until full dilation of the cervix.

The three phases of first stage labor are

a. Latent Phase
b. Active Phase
c. Transition Phase

Student Name Shirley Williams S.P.N.

15. The second stage of labor lasts from the time of full cervical dilation until the baby is birth.

16. The third stage of labor lasts from the birth of the baby until the placenta detaches & is expelled.

17. The fourth stage of labor is the first 1 to 4 hrs. following birth.

18. Describe typical maternal behaviors during each stage and phase of labor.

 a. First stage

 Latent phase Onset of labor until about 3 cm of cervical dilation, cervix effaces almost completely in the nullipara may remain thick in the multipara.

 Active phase Cervix dilates from 4 to 7 cm, effacement is completed. Membranes may rupture.

 Transition phase Cervix dilates from 8 to 10 cm. Intense contractions, firm 2-3 min. apart; duration ~~contraction~~ of some may be as long as 90 sec.

 b. Second stage Cervix fully dilated (10 cm) rectal pressure as fetus descends results in urge to push c contraction. (stage of expulsion)

 c. Third stage Woman may feel a slight cramp when placenta detaches uterus must contract firmly to control bleeding. (placental stage)

 d. Fourth stage uterus should remain firmly contracted about halfway between the woman's umbilicus & symphysis pubis (higher if infant was large) Bleeding (lochia rubra) should saturate no more than one pad/hour. (immediate postbirth recovery)

19. The normal fetal heart rate at term is ~~110~~ 120 at the lower limit and ~~150~~ 160 at the upper limit. The baseline rate usually fluctuates about 5 to 15 bpm.

20. a. Describe the appearance and odor of *normal* amniotic fluid.

 its clear + odorless

 b. Describe the appearance and odor of *abnormal* amniotic fluid.

 Green-stained, cloudy, or yellowish amniotic fluid + has a strong odor

21. Describe the assessments in the following categories that the nurse should promptly report when caring for a laboring woman.

    a. Temperature a temp. of 38°C (100.4°F)

    b. Blood pressure ____________________

    c. Fetal heart rate ____________________

22. What is the significance of the following patterns on the electronic fetal monitor? Include the nursing response to each, as appropriate.

    a. Variability Describes fluctuation, or constant changes in the base line rate.

    b. Accelerations are rate increases over the baseline rate of @ least 15 beats/min. lasting for @ least 15 seconds.

    c. Early decelerations are rate decreases during contractions; they always return to the baseline rate by the end of contractions.

    d. Variable decelerations begin + end abruptly; they are V-, W-, or U-shaped, they do not always exhibit a consistent pattern in relation to contraction

    e. Late decelerations look similar to early decelerations except that they do not return to the baseline FHR until after the contraction ends. late deceleration suggest that the placenta is not delivering enough oxygen to the fetus.

Student Name Shirley Williams S.P.N.

THINKING CRITICALLY

1. The following chart shows a typical status report often used in intrapartum units. Interpret the data about each woman's labor by answering the questions below.

Name	Gravida	Para	Gest	Dil	Eff	Sta	FHR
Amy	2	0	36	1–2	50%	–2	160
Becky	4	3	42	6	80%	–1	115
Cathy	1	0	40	3–4	90%	0	144
Deanna	3	1	39	C	C	+2	132

   a. Which client(s) is/are at full-term gestation?
   b. Which fetus(es) is/are engaged?
   c. Who is most likely to deliver first? Why?

2. What is the primary reason for observing the bladder closely immediately after birth? a full bladder inhibits uterine contraction and can lead to hemorrhage.

CASE STUDIES

1. A nurse working in a prenatal clinic must teach a woman when to go to the hospital. The woman is having her third baby. Her first labor lasted 18 hours and her second labor lasted 6 hours. What should the nurse teach this woman? Give a rationale for each part of your teaching.

2. A woman is in labor with her first baby. Her cervix is 7 cm dilated, and the fetal station is +1. Formulate appropriate nursing interventions for the nursing diagnosis Pain, related to labor process and exertion of labor.

OTHER LEARNING ACTIVITIES

1. Use a model of a pelvis and fetal head to place the head in each of the following positions. Move the head through each mechanism of labor for each of the positions.
   a. ROA
   b. ROT
   c. ROP
   d. LOA
   e. LOT
   f. LOP
   g. OA

2. During your clinical experience, note how different fetal presentations or positions affect the woman's comfort during labor. Note if there is an apparent effect on the length of labor.

3. Palpate the uterine contractions of women in labor and classify them as mild, moderate, or firm intensity. Confirm your observations with an experienced intrapartum nurse.

4. Observe the labor of a woman having a vaginal birth after cesarean (VBAC) for the following factors related to her experience.
   a. number of previous cesarean and vaginal births
   b. reason for previous cesarean birth
   c. the woman's desire to have this baby vaginally
   d. maternal behaviors during labor
   e. support of her partner
   f. her apparent feelings after birth, whether it was VBAC or a repeat cesarean

5. Examine electronic fetal monitor strips to identify the following features:
   a. information that the monitor automatically prints on the strip
   b. interface with computer device, if any
   c. differences in appearance between those obtained with external devices and those from internal devices
   d. presence or absence of variability, rate accelerations, and deceleration patterns
   e. nursing and medical responses to abnormal patterns; fetal response to interventions
   f. outcome of birth, including Apgar scores of the infant

6. Locate the "precip tray" in your clinical facility. What are the contents of this tray?

REVIEW QUESTIONS

1. During labor, a fetal heart rate of 125–135 bpm should be interpreted as
   a. probably normal.
   b. possibly abnormal.
   c. probably abnormal.
   d. clearly abnormal.

2. When assessing the duration of labor contractions, the nurse should time from the
   a. beginning of one contraction to the end of the same contraction.
   b. end of one contraction to the beginning of the next.
   c. beginning of one contraction to the beginning of the next.
   d. peak of one contraction to the peak of the next.

Student Name Shirley Williams S.P.N.

3. During normal labor, contractions characteristically become
   a. more frequent and of shorter duration.
   b. more frequent and of longer duration.
   c. less frequent and of shorter duration.
   d. less frequent and of longer duration.

4. When the fetus is in a cephalic presentation, the amniotic fluid is expected to be
   a. cloudy.
   b. clear.
   c. green.
   d. yellow.

5. The thinning of the cervix during labor is called
   a. dilation.
   b. effacement.
   c. station.
   d. presentation.

6. How should the nurse interpret the abbreviation ROP?
   a. The fetal sacrum is in the mother's right posterior pelvis.
   b. The fetal pelvis is in the mother's right occipital pelvis.
   c. The fetal occiput is in the mother's right posterior pelvis.
   d. The right fetal occiput is in the mother's posterior pelvis.

7. The labor phase when the woman often feels anxious, restless, and seems to lose control is
   a. latent.
   b. active.
   c. transition.
   d. placental.

8. Thirty minutes after birth, the nurse assesses the woman's uterine fundus. It is firm, above her umbilicus, and deviated to the right side. The appropriate nursing action is to
   a. massage the uterus.
   b. assist her to urinate.
   c. provide mild analgesia.
   d. restrict oral intake.

9. Choose the abbreviation that describes the fetus in a breech presentation.
   a. LSA.
   b. OA.
   c. ROA.
   d. LMT

10. Which sign or symptom normally occurs shortly before labor begins?
    a. an urge to push or bear down
    b. increased clear vaginal discharge
    c. moderate amount of vaginal bleeding
    d. sudden weight gain of 3–5 pounds

11. Fetal descent during labor is measured in relation to the mother's
    a. posterior perineum.
    b. sacral promontory.
    c. ischial spines.
    d. uterine fundus.

12. When the placenta is delivered with the fetal side presenting, the mechanism is called
    a. Duncan.
    b. Lamaze.
    c. VBAC.
    d. Schultze.

13. During the latent phase of labor, the nurse should expect the woman's behavior to be

    a. sleepy, except during contractions.

    b. mildly anxious, coping with contractions.

    c. quiet, concentrating on each contraction.

    d. frustrated, losing control with contractions.

14. A woman's membranes rupture during labor. The nurse notes that the fluid is yellowish and cloudy. The most important nursing response related to this assessment is to

    a. remove wet underpads and replace them with dry ones.

    b. perform a vaginal examination to assess labor progress.

    c. reassure the woman that membrane rupture is expected.

    d. assess the woman's temperature and the fetal heart rate.

15. The nurse should learn to evaluate labor progress by methods other than vaginal examination primarily because vaginal examination

    a. worsens the mother's discomfort.

    b. increases the risk for infection.

    c. reduces fetal heart rate variability.

    d. delays normal progression of labor.

16. Of those listed here, which is the most important nursing care during the second stage of labor?

    a. Observe the woman's perineum.

    b. Encourage pushing with contractions.

    c. Evaluate labor coping skills.

    d. Administer ordered analgesia.

17. Which maternal position should be *avoided* during labor?

    a. sitting

    b. walking

    c. side-lying

    d. supine

18. The woman having a vaginal birth after cesarean (VBAC) should be observed during labor particularly for signs of

    a. labor progression.

    b. uterine rupture.

    c. perineal pressure.

    d. excessive anxiety.

19. Which finding after nursing assessment should be promptly reported to the physician or nurse-midwife?

    a. clear amniotic fluid containing white flecks

    b. fetal heart rate of 144 bpm with variability

    c. vaginal discharge of mucus with dark blood

    d. contractions that last longer than 90 seconds

20. The priority nursing observation during the fourth stage is for

    a. vaginal bleeding.

    b. perineal bulging.

    c. uterine infection.

    d. parent-newborn bonding.

21. When assessing labor contractions, the nurse notes that the contracting uterus can be slightly indented with the fingertips when contractions are at their peak. Contraction intensity should be recorded as

    a. mild.

    b. moderate.

    c. firm.

    d. tetanic.

Student Name Shirley Williams S.P.N.

22. A woman phones the birth center and says, "I think my water broke, but I'm not having any contractions." The most appropriate nursing response is to tell her that
    a. labor should begin within a few hours at most.
    b. urine leakage is often confused with ruptured membranes.
    c. she should come to the birth center for evaluation.
    d. there is no concern unless the fluid is bloody.

23. Amniotic fluid usually turns Nitrazine paper
    a. yellow.
    b. green.
    c. dark blue.
    d. purple.

24. The nurse notes a pattern of variable decelerations on the electronic fetal monitor strip. The initial nursing response should be to
    a. reassure the woman that the pattern is expected.
    b. change the laboring woman's position.
    c. increase the rate of the nonadditive IV fluid.
    d. notify the physician of the abnormal pattern.

25. The primary means to identify hemorrhage after vaginal birth is to
    a. assess the vital signs frequently.
    b. observe the uterine fundus and lochia.
    c. keep an ice pack on the perineum.
    d. have the woman urinate every two hours.

chapter **7**

Nursing Management of Pain During Labor and Birth

LEARNING ACTIVITIES

1. Match the terms in the left column with their definitions on the right (a–e).

   C effleurage
   E endorphins
   D focal point
   A pain threshold
   B pain tolerance

   a. least amount of stimulation that a person perceives as painful
   b. maximum amount of pain one is willing to bear
   c. stroking of the abdomen, thighs, or other body parts
   d. intense concentration on an object
   e. internal substances similar to morphine

2. List four physical factors that cause pain during labor.
   a. C.N.S. Factors
   b. Maternal Condition
   c. Fetal Presentation + Position
   d. Interventions of Caregivers

3. How do each of these factors influence a woman's pain during labor?
   a. Cervical readiness Mother's cervix normally undergoes pre-labor changes that facilitate effacement and dilation in labor.
   b. Pelvic size and shape The size + shape of the pelvis significantly influence how readily the fetus can descend through it.

Student Name Shirly Williams S.P.N.

c. Labor intensity A woman who has a short intense labor often experiences more pain than the woman whose birth process is more gradual.

d. Maternal fatigue Fatigue reduces pain tolerance + a woman's ability to use coping skills.

e. Fetal presentation and position The fetal presenting part act as a wedge to efface + dilate the cervix as each contraction pushes it downward. Fetus abnormal presentation or position applies uneven pressure to the cervix, resulting in less effective effacement + dilation.

4. How does a woman's anxiety and fear relate to labor pain?

Excessive anxiety or fear raises her sensitivity to pain + reduces her ability to tolerate it.

5. List the benefits of each of these aspects of prenatal classes.

a. Education The woman who learns about changes during pregnancy and childbirth is less likely to respond c̄ fear + tension to labor.

b. Exercises Conditioning exercises, such as the pelvic rock, tailor sitting, and shoulder circling, prepare the woman's muscles for the demands of birth.

c. Relaxation techniques The laboring woman is guided to release the tension specifically, one muscle group @ a time, by saying "let your arms relax," let the tension out of your neck, your shoulder etc.

6. List three reasons why it is useful for any laboring woman to know nonpharmacologic pain control methods.

a. Nonpharmacologic methods help the woman to cope c̄ labor before it has advanced far enough to give her medication.

b. They do not slow labor if they provide adequate pain control. They carry no risk for allergy or adverse drug effects.

c. For best results, nonpharmacologic methods should be rehearsed before labor begins.

7. What nursing care may help a woman cope with the following problems during labor?

a. Hyperventilation Breathe slowly, especially in exhalation, breathe into cupped hands, breathe into small paper bag

b. Urge to push before complete cervical dilation The woman is taught to blow in short breaths to avoid bearing down. Pushing before full cervical dilation may cause cervical edema or lacerations.

8. Explain the differences between these anesthesia professionals.

   a. Anesthesiologist An anesthesiologist is a physician who specializes in giving anesthesia.

   b. Certified registered nurse-anesthetist (CRNA) is a registered nurse who has advanced training in anesthetic administration.

9. Explain why narcotic analgesics are usually not given if birth is expected within one hour of administration.

   The primary risk of narcotic analgesics is that they cross the placenta + can cause the infant's breathing @ birth to be sluggish.

10. What is the purpose of naloxone (Narcan)? What is an important nursing observation of the newborn related to use of this drug?

    is used to reverse respiratory depression. The nurse should observe for recurrent respiratory depression after each dose of naloxone until the depressant effects of the analgesic cease.

11. For each type of regional anesthetic listed below, describe (a) how it is administered, (b) the location of its pain relief, (c) its major side effects, and (d) medical and nursing measures related to its use.

Local infiltration

a. ~~Pudendal~~ injection of the ~~perineum~~ perineal ~~area~~ tissues

b. perineal ~~area~~ tissues are numbed.

c. There are virtually no risk if the woman is not allergic to the drug

d.

Student Name Shirley Williams S.P.N.

Pudendal block

a. The physician injects the pudendal nerves on each side of the mother's pelvis.

b. Perineum is also infiltrated because the pudendal block alone does not completely anesthetize the perineum

c. A vaginal hematoma or an abscess may develop, but this is not common

d.

Epidural block

a. The physician or nurse anesthetist penetrates the epidural space c̄ a large needle.

b. For cesarean birth numbness the woman's nipple level. For vaginal birth the level is about @ the hips.

c. Long ~~term~~ ~~respir~~ acting epidural narcotics can cause respiratory depression that may occur many hrs. after they are injected

d. The nurse should palpate the bladder 2 hours or more often if a large quantity of IV solution was given.

Intrathecal analgesics

a. Injection of opiod analgesics into the sub-arachnoid space.

b. Intrathecal analgesics do not produce the anesthesia needed for surgical procedures.

c. Limited duration of action, inadequate pain relief for late labor + the birth itself

d. Observe for late occurring respiratory depression. Naloxone should be readily available. N/V + itching may occur.

Subarachnoid block

a. injected into the dura mater c̄ a thin 25 to 27 gauge spinal needle.

b. The woman loses movement and sensation below the block

c. Hypotension and urinary retention are the main adverse effects.

d. Bedrest, analgesics + oral + intravenous fluids, a blood patch done by the nurse-anesthetist or anesthesiologist.

12. An anesthesiologist gives a test dose of the anesthetic agent when starting an epidural block to identify if the catheter is in the right place. The expected reaction to the test dose is numbness or loss of movement.

13. The woman who plans to have epidural anesthesia during labor and birth should be particularly questioned about allergy to Dental anesthetics.

14. What is potentially the most life-threatening complication of general anesthesia for the mother? What is done to reduce the risk?

Regurgitation c̄ aspiration (breathing in) of the acidic stomach contents; result in aspiration pneumonitis can be fatal. Several drugs are used to reduce gastric acidity, an oral antacid, such as sodium citrate c̄ citric acid (Bicitra), 15mL.

Student Name Sharif William S.P.N.

THINKING CRITICALLY

1. Why do you think general anesthesia is rarely used for vaginal delivery?

CASE STUDIES

1. a. Jill Sims is a primigravida in labor at 4 cm cervical dilation. She is using breathing techniques she learned in prepared childbirth classes. Jill is breathing rapidly throughout each contraction. She complains of stiff fingers and numbness around her mouth. What is the probable cause of Jill's symptoms? What is an appropriate nursing measure to help correct her problem?

   b. Jill is now 5–6 cm dilated and requests an epidural block. Is this an appropriate time during labor to give an epidural block? If so, what nursing observations are most important after the block is begun?

   c. What nursing measures are appropriate during second-stage labor?

2. You are working with a laboring woman and note that she is holding her body stiffly and gripping the bed rails tightly during each contraction. What nursing interventions are appropriate in each of the following areas?
   a. relaxation techniques
   b. adjusting the environment
   c. assisting her with breathing techniques

OTHER LEARNING ACTIVITIES

1. When you are in the hospital, look at trays used to administer various anesthetics. Identify the following components in the trays.
   a. pudendal block tray: Iowa trumpet
   b. epidural block tray: Touhy needle, epidural catheter
   c. subarachnoid (spinal) block tray: spinal needle (note the size difference from the epidural needle)
2. Identify professionals in your hospital who administer obstetrical anesthesia. Are they limited to administration of specific types of anesthesia? Is one present 24 hours a day? Do obstetricians give epidural blocks?
3. Look at the contents of emergency carts for women and newborns. Who usually handles emergency care of newborns who are in distress? Do they hold certification from the American Heart Association and American Academy of Pediatrics in neonatal resuscitation?
4. What is the most common anesthesia for vaginal birth in your hospital? For cesarean birth?
5. Observe a childbirth education class.
6. Observe a laboring woman using childbirth preparation techniques. Who is her support person? How is the support person helping her use these techniques? How can you help her?

REVIEW QUESTIONS

1. According to the gate control theory, which technique should be most helpful in interrupting transmission of labor pain to the brain?

   a. rapid, shallow breathing

   b. application of heat

   c. focusing on a point in the room

   d. deep cleansing breaths

2. The primary purpose of Kegel exercises is to

   a. increase skeletal flexibility.

   b. relieve back discomfort.

   c. promote body relaxation.

   d. strengthen pelvic muscles.

3. Butorphanol differs from meperidine in that butorphanol

   a. can interfere with pure narcotics.

   b. causes greater respiratory depression.

   c. completely eliminates labor pain.

   d. cannot be reversed with naloxone.

4. The newborn of a woman who receives narcotic analgesics during labor should be observed for

   a. convulsions.

   b. slow respirations.

   c. excess activity.

   d. constipation.

5. A woman (gravida 2, para 1) plans an epidural block for labor and birth. Which factor in her history is most significant in terms of her planned anesthetic?

   a. mild hypertension during first pregnancy

   b. light meal four hours before labor began

   c. forceps delivery during first birth

   d. adverse reaction to dental anesthetic

6. An advantage of an epidural block is that it

   a. reduces pain for both labor and birth.

   b. has no fetal or maternal risks.

   c. supports normal blood pressure.

   d. enhances the woman's urge to push.

7. Immediately after birth, nursing care for the woman who had subarachnoid block anesthesia for a repeat cesarean birth should include

   a. ambulating within two hours of birth.

   b. keeping her back curved outward.

   c. assessing for return of sensation.

   d. keeping her flat in bed for eight hours.

8. A blood patch may be done to relieve

   a. low blood pressure.

   b. respiratory depression.

   c. postspinal headache.

   d. prolonged numbness.

Student Name S. Riley Williams S.b.N.

9. The nurse should observe the woman who received epidural narcotics for

a. late respiratory depression.

b. nausea and vomiting.

c. unstable blood pressure.

d. persistent headache.

10. Sodium citrate with citric acid (Bicitra) is given to

a. reduce gastric acidity.

b. prevent pulmonary aspiration.

c. promote respiratory function.

d. increase maternal blood pressure.

11. During general anesthesia, cricoid pressure is done to

a. reduce stomach acid secretion.

b. avoid aspiration of gastric contents.

c. prevent excessive blood loss.

d. prevent musculoskeletal injuries.

12. A woman asks if she should take prepared childbirth classes. The best response of the nurse is to tell her that classes will

a. allow her to avoid pain medications during labor.

b. be required if her partner wants to be with her.

c. provide methods to help her cope with labor.

d. reduce the likelihood that complications will occur.

13. The prepared childbirth technique that is most likely to relieve back pain during labor is

a. effleurage.

b. sacral pressure.

c. distraction.

d. patterned breathing.

14. A woman is using prepared childbirth breathing techniques and complains of dizziness and tingling. The nurse should

a. have her breathe more rapidly with contractions.

b. ask her if she feels an urge to push or bear down.

c. tell her to breathe slowly into her cupped hands.

d. reassure her that these sensations are normal.

15. A possible risk of prolonged pushing while holding the breath during second stage labor is that it

a. may result in a too-rapid birth.

b. can decrease fetal oxygenation.

c. results in maternal exhaustion.

d. increases uterine blood supply.

16. Immediately after an epidural block is begun, the woman should be positioned

a. flat on her back, with no pillow.

b. sitting upright with her legs over the side of the bed.

c. with a small roll under her right hip.

d. in a modified Trendelenburg position.

17. The most common purpose of naltrexone (Trexan) in maternity care is to

a. relieve early postpartum pain.

b. limit gastric acid production.

c. decrease pruritus (itching).

d. enhance the effects of narcotics.

18. An appropriate independent nursing measure to help reduce a postspinal headache is to
    a. encourage increased oral fluid intake.
    b. position with the head elevated.
    c. provide analgesics around the clock.
    d. reduce position changes in bed.

19. Two hours after a vaginal birth with an epidural anesthesia, the nurse determines that the woman's bladder is full. The most appropriate initial nursing action is to
    a. help her walk to the bathroom to urinate.
    b. evaluate movement and sensation of her legs.
    c. insert an indwelling (Foley) catheter.
    d. take no action at this time.

20. The most effective way to identify adequate maternal oxygenation after general anesthesia for cesarean birth is to
    a. take the blood pressure regularly.
    b. observe for cyanosis or restlessness.
    c. maintain a side-lying position.
    d. observe pulse-oximeter readings.

Student Name [illegible]

chapter **8**

Nursing Care of Women with Complications During Labor and Birth

LEARNING ACTIVITIES

1. Match the terms in the left column with their definitions on the right (a–h).

F	amniotomy	a.	infection of the amniotic sac
G	cephalopelvic disproportion	b.	excessive amniotic fluid
D	chignon	c.	substance that swells within the cervix, dilating it slightly
A	chorioamnionitis	d.	circular swelling on the neonate's head caused by vacuum extractor
H	dystocia	e.	large body size
B	hydramnios	f.	artificial rupture of the amniotic sac
C	laminaria	g.	inability of the fetus to fit through the pelvis
E	macrosomia	h.	difficult labor

2. Describe three potential complications of amniotomy and the nursing assessments that should be reported for each.

a. Prolapse of the umbilical cord
Infection
Abruptio Placentae

b. Identifying Complication, the FHR is recorded for @ least 1 min, a large quantity of fluid increases the risk for prolapsed cord,

c. The color, odor, amount & character of amniotic fluid are recorded. The woman's temp. is taken q 2 to 4 hrs. Meconium-stained amniotic fluid.

3. Distinguish between labor *induction* and labor *augmentation*.
Induction of labor the initiation of labor before it begins naturally. Augmentation is the stimulation of contractions after they have begun naturally.

4. Identify each drug or class of drugs from the following descriptions of their main purpose.
   a. Soften the cervix Prostaglandin in the form of a gel or a commercially prepared vaginal insert.
   b. Stimulate labor contractions Oxytocin initiation or stimulation of contraction.
   c. Inhibit uterine contractions Tocolytic drugs may be given.
   d. Speed fetal lung maturation Dexamethasone and betamethasone are two drugs for this purpose.

5. Describe three nursing measures to promote comfort in a woman who has an episiotomy or perineal laceration.
   a. Cold application + analgesics
   b. Warmth in the form of heat packs
   c. Sitz bath

6. Two separate incisions are done in cesarean delivery. What are they? Which of the two is more important and why? Two types of cesarean incisions are skin incision + uterine incision - the more important of the two incision is the one that cuts into the uterus.

7. What nursing observations are appropriate after cesarean birth in each of the following areas?
   a. IV - site and rate ~~and~~ of solution flow
   b. Uterine fundus for firmness, height, and midline position.

Student Name Shirly Williams S.P.N.

c. Dressing for drainage .

d. Lochia for quantity, color and presence of clots

e. Indwelling catheter urine output.

8. Compare *hypotonic* labor to *hypertonic* labor for the following characteristics.

a. Contractions hypotonic labor contraction are too weak to be effective + hypertonic labor contraction are frequent, cramplike & poorly coordinated.

b. Time of occurrence during labor hypotonic The woman begins labor normally, but contraction diminsh during the active phase (after 4cm of cervical dilation, when the pace of labor is expected to accelerate. Hypertonic labor usually occurs during the latent phase of labor (before 4cm of cervial dilation) It is less common hypotonic dysfunction.

c. Medical management Hypotonic labor the physician usually does an amniotomy if the membranes are intact. Augmentation of labor c̄ oxytocin or by nipple stimulation ↑ the strength of contraction.
Hypertonic labor mild sedation to allow the woman to rest. Tocolytic drugs such as terbutaline (Brenthine), may be order to reduce ↑ uterine resting tone.

d. Nursing care Hypotonic labor - in addion to providing care R/t amniotomy + labor augmentation, the nurse gives emotional support to the woman and her partner. Position changes may help to relieve discomfort + enhance progress.
Hypertonic labor - the women are uncomfortable + frustrated. The nurse should accept the woman's frustration and that of her partner. The nurse provides general comfort measures that promote rest and relaxation.

9. Describe how each of the following factors can contribute to abnormal labor and list nursing measures appropriate for each.

   a. Ineffective pushing efforts because she does not understand which tech. to use or she fears tearing her perineal tissues. Epidural or subarachnoid block may depress the urge to push. Nursing care - focus on coaching the woman about the most effective tech. for pushing. If she cannot feel her contractions because of a regional block, the nurse tells her when to push.

   b. Occiput posterior fetal position Most women c̄ an average-size pelvis cannot deliver the infant who remain in an occiput posterior position. During labor the nurse should encourage the woman to assume positions that favor fetal rotation & descent. These positions also reduce some of the back pain. Good positions for back labor include the following:

10. Explain how excessive psychologic stress can contribute to a difficult labor.

    If their stress is too high, however, they perceive more pain & often have inadequate contractions. Their body responds to stress c̄ a "fight-or-flight" reaction.

11. Describe four possible adverse effects of prolonged labor on either the mother or the fetus. Maternal or newborn infection, especially if the membranes have been ruptured for a long time.

    a.

    b. Maternal exhaustion

    c. Postpartum hemorrhage

    d. Greater anxiety & fear in an ensuing pregnancy

12. Explain the difference between precipitous *labor* and precipitous *birth*.

    Precipitous labor is completed in less than 3 hrs. Precipitate birth is one that occurs unexpectedly, c̄ no trained birth attendant present.

Student Name Shirley Williams S.P.N.

13. Describe possible adverse effects of precipitous labor on the mother and fetus.

a. Fetal oxygenation can be compromised by intense contraction

b. She may have uterine rupture, cervical lacerations or hematoma.

c. Birth injury from rapid passage through the birth canal may become evident in the infant after birth. These injuries can include intracranial hemorrhage or nerve damage.

14. What is the difference between PROM and PPROM?

Premature rupture of the membranes (PROM) Rupture of the membranes @ term 38 or more wks gestation before labor. Preterm Premature rupture of the membranes (PPROM) rupture of the membranes before term (38 wks gestation) c or s uterine contractions.

15. What is the role of each of the following measures in the care of the woman with threatened or actual preterm labor?

a. Activity restrictions The initial measures to stop preterm labor include identifying + treating infection, activity restriction.

b. Fetal fibronectin helps the physician decide which women should be treated most aggressively to stop preterm labor.

c. Urinalysis Urinary tract infections increase the risk for preterm labor + birth, so urinalysis is done.

16. List three nursing observations of the fetus or neonate when pregnancy is prolonged.

a. Observe the fetus during labor to identify signs associated c poor placental blood flow, such as late decelerations.

b. After birth, the newborn is observe for respiratory difficulties.

c. Hypoglycemia.

17. List four situations in which the nurse must be especially watchful for a prolapsed umbilical cord.

    a. Fetus high in the pelvis when the membranes rupture.

    b. Very small fetus, as in prematurity.

    c. abnormal presentation, such as footling breech or transverse lie

    d. Hydramnios (excess amniotic fluid)

18. Describe three variations of uterine rupture. Which is the most common?

    a. Complete rupture - a hole thru the uterine wall from the uterine cavity to the abdominal cavity.

    b. Incomplete rupture - uterus tears into a nearby structure such as a ligament, but not all the way into the abdominal cavity.

    c. Dehiscence - an old uterine scar, usually from a previous cesarean birth separates; the separation may be bloodless.

THINKING CRITICALLY

1. In addition to assessing the progress of labor, what other nursing assessments are important for the woman who has a precipitous labor? How can positioning the woman on her side improve the fetus's oxygen supply?

   assess FHT. reposition pt. on L side relieve the pressure

CASE STUDIES

1. Cara Miller is a 24-year-old gravida 2, para 1, who is in early labor with her first baby. Her cervix is 3 cm dilated and 75% effaced; fetal station is 0. Contractions are every 4 minutes, 30–35 seconds in duration, and of moderate intensity. The nurse-midwife performs an amniotomy. A small amount of light-green fluid drains on the underpad.

    a. Use your birth facility's standard form to chart this information about Cara's labor.

    b. What nursing interventions are appropriate now?

    c. Is there any significance to the color of the amniotic fluid? If so, what is the significance?

    d. Describe observations that would suggest that the amniotomy caused complications.

Student Name Shirley Williams S.P.N.

2. Baby boy Briggs was born in a forceps-assisted birth. What observations should the nurse make in each area listed below?

a. skin Examined for lacerations, abrasions or bruising.

b. shape of head - mild facial redding & molding of the head are common & require no treatment.

c. appearance when crying

3. Write a simple explanation to parents about the infant's head shape after a forceps birth. Reassure them that they are temporary and usually resolve ~~without~~ without treatment.

OTHER LEARNING ACTIVITIES

1. Observe newborns who were in abnormal presentations or positions before birth. Identify characteristics caused by the abnormal presentation or position.

2. What interventions do nurses in your clinical setting use when a mother is having complicated labor? How did you contribute to a mother's physical or psychologic comfort during labor? What was the reason for the woman's abnormal labor?

3. What drugs to stop preterm labor are prescribed in your clinical setting? Read the policies and procedures related to administration of the drugs. If possible, assist in the care of a woman who is receiving the drugs. What concerns do the woman and her family share with the staff?

4. Visit a service that provides home nursing care to women at risk for preterm labor or with other complications of pregnancy. What care do nurses provide?

5. Make a list of activities appropriate for a woman on activity restriction for preterm labor, both in the hospital and at home.

6. Observe a woman who has a cesarean birth after labor, focusing on her feelings about the surgical birth. Compare your observations with those of classmates who have cared for other women who had cesarean births.

REVIEW QUESTIONS

1. After amniotomy, which of the following observations should be reported immediately?

a. clear fluid draining on the underpad

b. maternal temperature of 37.2°C (99.0°F)

(c.) fetal heart rate of 95 bpm

d. moderate contractions every three minutes

2. Which is the most appropriate nursing care for the woman having hypertonic labor?

a. Encourage walking in the hallway.

(b.) Promote rest and general comfort.

c. Give her simple foods and liquids.

d. Limit oral and intravenous fluids.

3. A woman, gravida 4, para 3, has been 5 cm dilated for 2 hours. Her contractions are every 7 minutes, 30 seconds duration, and mild. The FHR is 135–145/minute. She is relatively comfortable. This woman is most likely experiencing
   a. hypotonic labor dysfunction.
   b. hypertonic labor dysfunction.
   c. occiput posterior fetal position.
   d. fetal shoulder dystocia.

4. The most desirable position for a woman having a precipitous labor is
   a. side-lying.
   b. semi-Fowler's.
   c. Trendelenburg.
   d. hands and knees.

5. After a vaginal birth complicated by shoulder dystocia, the nurse should particularly assess the newborn for
   a. molding of the head.
   b. flexed positioning.
   c. clavicle deformity.
   d. abnormal temperature.

6. A woman has ruptured membranes at 35 weeks gestation. Which nursing observation should be promptly reported?
   a. FHR averages 145–150 bpm
   b. occasional mild contractions
   c. spontaneous fetal movement
   d. temperature of 38.2°C (100.8°F)

7. Which is the most typical labor characteristic when the fetus is in an occiput posterior position?
   a. labor length under three hours
   b. persistent back discomfort
   c. rapid fetal descent
   d. mild contraction strength

8. A woman who is at 32 weeks gestation telephones the nurse in a labor unit and says that her baby seems to be "pushing down" much of the time and that she has a constant backache. Choose the most appropriate nursing response.
   a. Ask her to have someone bring her to the labor unit for further assessment.
   b. Reassure her that pressure and backache are common during late pregnancy.
   c. Tell her she should rest with her feet elevated several times each day.
   d. Encourage her to promote bladder emptying by increasing her fluid intake.

9. External version is most likely to be done in which of these situations?
   a. early labor with frank breech presentation
   b. breech presentation with placenta previa
   c. twins in cephalic and breech presentations
   d. breech presentation at 38 weeks gestation

10. The first nursing action for a visibly prolapsed umbilical cord is to
   a. call the physician or nurse-midwife.
   b. palpate the cord for a pulse.
   c. apply the internal fetal monitor.
   d. relieve pressure on the cord.

11. What is the priority nursing action following amniotomy?
   a. Turn the woman to her side.
   b. Check the fetal heart rate.
   c. Assess the color of the fluid.
   d. Change the underpad.

Student Name ___________________________

12. The nursing intervention most likely to make the woman with a perineal laceration more comfortable during the first two hours after birth is

    a. warm water soaks.
    b. a small dressing.
    c. an ice pack.
    d. antibacterial ointment.

13. The parents of a newborn delivered with low forceps ask about small bruises on each side of the baby's head. The nurse should tell the parents that the bruises

    a. will be reported to the physician.
    b. usually disappear in a few days.
    c. may indicate brain damage.
    d. occur in all deliveries.

14. The most important nursing care during the recovery period after cesarean birth is to

    a. provide analgesia.
    b. assess the fundus.
    c. position for comfort.
    d. encourage urination.

15. When caring for a woman after a car accident during the third trimester of pregnancy, the nurse should observe the fetus primarily for signs of

    a. undetected trauma.
    b. poor oxygenation.
    c. intrauterine infection.
    d. preterm birth.

16. The nurse must particularly observe for signs and symptoms of uterine rupture if the laboring woman has

    a. a hypotonic labor pattern.
    b. a prior cesarean birth.
    c. prematurely ruptured membranes.
    d. a large fetus.

17. An infant's amniotic fluid was meconium stained. During the admission assessment, the nurse notes that the infant's skin is peeling and that she has a long, thin appearance. These facts suggest that this infant is probably

    a. preterm.
    b. postterm.
    c. hypoglycemic.
    d. anemic.

18. A woman has prostaglandin gel applied to her cervix the day before she is scheduled for induction of labor. Which is the most appropriate teaching before she returns home?

    a. Do not eat or drink anything until you return for labor induction.
    b. Your bag of waters will probably rupture before you return tomorrow.
    c. Return to the birth center if you begin having regular contractions.
    d. Stay in bed, lying on your left side, until you return for labor induction.

19. An infant is born by elective (planned) cesarean birth because of a breech presentation. The infant weighs 7 pounds, 1 ounce (3,206 g). The nursery nurse should particularly observe this infant for

    a. low blood sugar.
    b. respiratory difficulty.
    c. birth injury.
    d. generalized infection.

chapter **9**

The Family After Birth

LEARNING ACTIVITIES

1. Match the terms in the left column with their definitions on the right (a–f).

D	atony	a.	top of the uterus
B	colostrum	b.	first breast secretion after birth
A	fundus	c.	vaginal drainage after birth
F	involution	d.	lack of muscle tone
C	lochia	e.	first six weeks after birth
E	puerperium	f.	return of the uterus to its normal state after birth

2. Describe the following expected assessments for the uterine fundus immediately after birth.

   a. Location Between the mother's umbilicus and symphysis.

   b. Consistency firmness

3. Describe the initial nursing action if the fundus is boggy (soft) and bleeding is excessive during the postpartum period. How does this action control uterine bleeding?

   if the mother fundus is soft, massage it (supporting the lower segment) the expel clots so it will remain contracted. If the bladder is also full, massage the uterus until firm, then address emptying the bladder. Control bleeding first, then keep it control by emptying the bladder

4. List two drugs that may be ordered to correct uterine atony.

   a. Methylergonovine maleate (methergine)

   b. Oxytocin (Pitocin Syntocinon)

Student Name Shirley Williams S.P.N.

5. List and describe the three stages of lochia.

a. lochia rubra - It is composed of endometrial tissue, blood, and lymph.

b. Lochia serosa - is pinkish because of its blood + mucus content. It lasts from 3rd - 10th day after birth

c. lochia alba - is mostly mucus + is clear + colorless or white. it lasts from the 10th - 14th day after birth.

6. When should perineal care be done?

a. After each voiding or bowel movement.

b. And ~~after~~ during changing of each pad.

7. What should the nurse teach a postpartum woman about applying and removing her perineal pad?

Perineal pads should be applied + removed in the same front-to-back direction to prevent fecal contamination of the perineum + vagina

8. The new mother can expect her menstrual periods to resume in 6 to 8 weeks if she is not breastfeeding, and in 2 to 18 months if she is breastfeeding.

9. Average blood loss at birth is about 500 mL for vaginal birth and 1000 mL for cesarean birth.

10. Describe two nursing actions that may make a woman who is chilled and shaking after birth more comfortable.

a. a warm blanket

b. a warm ~~drink~~ Drink

11. Describe three possible signs of a full bladder in the immediate postpartum period.

a. Height of uterus uterus is high

b. Location of uterus deviates to one side (right)

c. Uterine tone __________

12. Describe three nursing actions that may help a new mother to empty her bladder after birth.

    a. Provide as much privacy as possible

    b. Run water in the sink

    c. Have her place her hands in warm H_2O.

13. Nursing measures to prevent or correct constipation after birth include

    a. Encourage to drink lots of fluids

    b. Add fiber to her diet & ambulate

    c. A stool softener is usually ordered

14. Describe each of the following factors about postbirth use of Rh_o(D) immune globulin (Rh_oGAM).

    a. Mother's Rh factor negative

    b. Infant's Rh factor positive

    c. Recommended time of administration 72 hrs after birth

    d. Site and route of administration intramuscular (deltoid) injection.

15. Explain each of the following factors about postpartum rubella immunization.

    a. Why it is given to the nonimmune woman at this time The vaccine prevents infection c̄ the rubella virus during subsequent pregnancies, which could cause birth defects.

    b. Common reactions Mild symptoms of rubella, such as rash, malaise, sore throat, headache, joint pain & slight fever.

    c. Precautions Do not administer the vaccine if she is sensitive to neomycin or if she has had a transfusion within the last 3 months.

16. What assessments should the nurse make in each of these areas when caring for the woman who has had a cesarean birth?

    a. Bleeding The quantity of lochia is generally less after cesarean birth

    b. Uterine fundus If the fundus is firm & @ its expected level no massage is necessary.

    c. Urinary output Measure the first 2 to 3 voidings, or until the woman urinates @ least 150 mL.

Student Name Shirley Williams S.P.N.

17. Name and describe Rubin's three postpartum psychologic phases.

a. Phase 1 - Mother is passive and willing (taking in) to let others do for her

b. Phase 2 - Taking hold - Mother begins to initiate action + becomes interested in caring for baby.

c. Phase 3 - letting go - Mothers, and often fathers, work through giving up their previous life style + family arrangements to incorporate the new infant.

18. a. Describe postpartum blues. A new mothers often experience conflicting feeling of joy + emotional let down during the first few weeks after birth.

b. What are the appropriate nursing interventions for this emotional reaction?

19. Describe nursing interventions that may be appropriate for grieving families in the maternity setting.

The nurse should listen to them + support them. Therapeutic communication tech. such as open-ended questions or reflecting feeling help the parents to express their grief an early step in resolving it

20. List five observations that suggest abnormal newborn respiratory function.

a. Cyanosis, other than of the hands + feet

b. Grunting respiration, which may be audible only c̄ a stethoscope

c. Retraction of the abdomen under the ribs

d. Flaring of the nostrils

e. Sustained, respiratory rate higher than 60 breath/min.

21. List four perinatal factors that should alert the nurse to the newborn's possible need for resuscitation.

    a. Heart Rate

    b. Respiratory Effort

    c. Skin Color

    d. Reflex Response to suction or a gentle slap on the soles

22. The drug used to reverse narcotic-induced respiratory depression in the newborn is Narcan (Naloxone).

23. Assign an Apgar score to each of the following newborns and briefly define what this score means in each case.

    a. Heart rate 110; slow breathing; some flexion of extremities; cries when stimulated; body pink, extremities bluish.

       2-

    b. Heart rate 135; crying at intervals; actively moves all extremities; coughs when suctioned; body pink, extremities bluish.

       2

    c. Heart rate 85; slow, irregular breathing; flaccid muscle tone; grimaces when suctioned; color blue.

       1

24. Why is prevention of neonatal hypothermia particularly important?

    Newborn infant has less efficient means of generating heat than an older infant. hypothermia can cause hypoglycemia + respiratory distress.

25. Describe why and how the nurse uses each of these methods to reduce neonatal heat loss.

    a. Drying

    b. Hat

    c. Radiant warmer a skin probe is placed over the infant liver or spleen area (right or left abdomen) to act as a thermostat ↑ or ↓ heat output from the radiant

    d. Parental contact Place infant in skin-to-skin contact c̄ a parent.

Student Name Shirley Williams S.P.N.

26. Match the routes of neonatal heat loss with the situations on the right (a–d) in which they are most likely to occur.

A evaporation	a. air-conditioning vent blowing air on infant.
B conduction	b. infant placed on cool padded surface for assessment.
C convection	c. parents bathing infant slowly.
D radiation	d. infant's crib located near a window on a cold day.

27. The nurse should normally be able to identify how many arteries in the newborn's umbilical cord? two How many veins? one

28. Why are most newborns given vitamin K after birth?

Vit. K is necessary to form several coagulation factors (VII, IX, X). One dose of vit. K, 0.5 to 1mg, is given in an intra-muscular (IM) injection to give the baby the vit. until their intestinal bacteria produce it.

29. a. The newborn's eyes should be treated after birth to prevent what disorder?

Gonorrhea & Chlamydia

b. This disorder is caused by what organisms?

c. What is the most common medication to prevent the disorder?

Erythromycin ointment

30. List seven common laboratory screening tests for newborns. Identify the one that is mandatory in all states.

a. Phenylketonuria (PKU) is mandatory in all states
b. hypothyroidism
c. galactosemia
d. Sickle cell disease
e. Thalassemia
f. Maple syrup urine disease
g. Homocystinuria

31. Describe the newborn's first and second periods of reactivity.

    a. First begin @ birth, the infant is awake, alert & seems to enjoy gazing @ the surrounding.

    b. Second after a deep sleep of 2 to 4 hrs, the baby is more interested in feeding & may pass the first meconium stool.

32. List three types of parent-infant contact that enhance attachment. Which of these is most important?

    a. __________

    b. __________

    c. __________

33. Describe the actions of hormones that are important in lactation.

    a. Prolactin from the anterior pituitary gland, which causes the manufacture of breast milk.

    b. Oxytocin from the posterior pituitary gland, which cause milk to be delivered from the alveoli (milk-producing sacs)

34. a. Describe colostrum.

    it high in protein content, provides some immune properties & cleanses the newborn's intestinal tract of mucus & meconium.

    b. Explain the neonatal benefits of colostrum.

    It aids in eliminates meconium

35. Describe breast engorgement and methods to relieve it. The breast & areola are very tense & distended, the mother can pump her breasts to get the milk flow started & soften the areola.

36. Describe the following nutritional needs of the breastfeeding mother.

    a. Calories 500 additional calories each day

    b. Foods meat, fish, poultry, eggs, beans & nuts

    c. Fluids 8 to 10 glasses of H_2O a day

    d. Vitamins continue prenatal vitamins

Student Name Shirley Williams S.N.

37. What should the nurse teach the breastfeeding mother in each of the following areas?

a. Foods that the infant may not tolerate Chocolate, cabbage, beans + broccoli.

b. Smoking Cigarette smoking exposes the infant to nicotine + may reduce milk production.

c. Alcohol Can interfere c̄ the let-down reflex + may be harmful to the infant.

d. Medications In general, if a medication can be taken by a newborn, it is safe to be taken by a lactating woman.

38. List four forms of infant formula.

a. Similac + Enfamil

b. Ready-to-feed, either in can or in glass bottles

c. Concentrated liquid formula

d. Powdered formula

39. Describe teaching in each of the following areas for bottle-feeding parents.

a. Propping the bottle

b. Nipple positioning in mouth

c. Microwaving is not recommended. The center becomes very hot in a microwave although the outside is cool.

d. Burping about 1/2 to 1 oz. @ first, gradually increasing the amount between burps as the stomach capacity enlarges.

e. Positioning baby after feeding Slightly elevating the upper body @ the end of the feeding reduces regurgitation.

f. Leftover formula Should be discarded as microorganisms from the mouth grow rapidly in warm formula.

40. Describe appropriate nursing teaching in the following areas for postpartum discharge.

a. Rest Avoid strenuous activity + do no heavy lifting, napping when the baby is napping.

b. Hygiene A daily shower or bath is refreshing, Perineal care should be continued until lochia stops.

c. Sexual intercourse Coitus should be avoided until the episiotomy is fully healed & the lochia flow has stopped.

d. Exercise ______________________________

e. Diet A well balanced diet promotes healing & recovery from birth.

41. List nine danger signals that a postpartum woman should promptly report to her physician or nurse-midwife.

a. Fever higher than 38°C (100.4°F)
b. Persistent lochia rubra or lochia that has a foul odor
c. Bright red bleeding, particularly if lochia has change to serosa or alba
d. Prolonged afterpains, pelvic or abdominal pain or a constant backache.
e. Signs of urinary tract infection, previously described.
f. Pain, redness, or tenderness of the calf
g. localized breast tenderness or redness
h. Discharge, pain, redness, or separation of any suture line (cesarean, perineal laceration or episiotomy)
i. Prolonged & pervasive feeling of depression or being let down; generally not enjoying life.

THINKING CRITICALLY

1. After a cesarean birth, what are some nursing interventions to help a mother manage pain while remaining alert enough to nurse her baby? Why is this mother likely to need additional nutrition teaching?

CASE STUDY

1. a. Cynthia Chung, 26 years old, is expecting her first baby in about 12 weeks. She says that she is having a difficult time deciding whether to breastfeed or bottle feed her baby. What information should you provide Cynthia to help her make this decision? What information would be available to use at your clinical facility?

   b. Cynthia decides to breastfeed her baby. On the third day after birth, she phones the unit to say that she has breast engorgement and her nipples are sore. Her left nipple has a small crack. What can the nurse teach Cynthia to help her cope with these problems?

   c. What should the nurse teach Cynthia about care of the baby's umbilical stump? What signs of problems should she report?

Student Name Shirley Williams S.P.N.

OTHER LEARNING ACTIVITIES

1. What analgesics do postpartum women in your hospital receive for pain? Do nurses use any nonpharmacologic techniques to make the women more comfortable?

2. Assess newborns in the delivery room for Apgar scores. How do your Apgar scores compare with the staff nurse's scores? What actions are taken for Apgar scores lower than 7 at 1 minute of age?

3. Is certification in the Neonatal Resuscitation Program required of nurses who work in the delivery room and nursery of your hospital?

4. What drug for newborn eye care does your hospital use? Observe newborns for side effects from or reactions to the drugs used.

5. Observe families during the postpartum period. What interactions do you see between mother, father, and newborn? Identify practices in your clinical setting that enhance or inhibit parent-infant attachment.

6. Assist the staff nurse to help new mothers learn to breastfeed. If you have successfully breastfed a baby yourself, share appropriate helpful hints with new mothers and classmates.

REVIEW QUESTIONS

1. Which of the following postpartum patient assessments requires immediate nursing intervention?
   a. excretion of large amounts of urine on first postpartum day
   b. soft fundus, to right of the midline, two hours after birth
   c. nipples intact but reddened on the first postpartum day
   d. perineal area edematous and tender, with slight bruising

2. The most serious potential problem if a woman's bladder is distended in the early postpartum period is
   a. infection.
   b. discomfort.
   c. vomiting.
   d. hemorrhage.

3. Which of these women is most likely to have afterpains?
   a. gravida 1, para 1, 6.5 lb (2,951 g) infant
   b. gravida 3, para 1, 7 lb (3,178 g) infant
   c. gravida 1, para 1, twins weighing 3.5 lb (1,589 g) and 4.5 lb (2,043 g)
   d. gravida 4, para 4, 9.5 lb (4,313 g) infant

4. Two hours after a woman's uncomplicated vaginal birth requiring no anesthesia, the nurse notes that her uterus is firm, two fingerwidths above her umbilicus, and deviated slightly to her right side. The most appropriate nursing action at this time is to
   a. check her blood pressure and pulse.
   b. massage her uterus continuously.
   c. insert an indwelling catheter.
   d. help her walk to the bathroom to urinate.

5. Choose the situation that describes appropriate administration of Rh_o(D) immune globulin (Rh_oGAM).

   a. Rh-negative infant, Rh-negative mother, given IV to the infant within 12 hours of birth

   b. Rh-positive infant, Rh-negative mother, given IV to the mother within one week of birth

   c. Rh-positive infant, Rh-negative mother, given IM to the mother within 72 hours of birth

   d. Rh-negative infant, Rh-positive mother, given IM to the mother within 72 hours of birth

6. When teaching parents about PKU testing, the nurse should teach them that

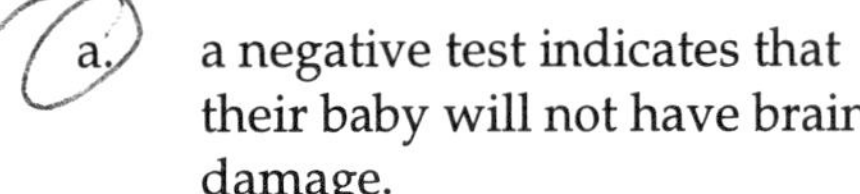

   a. a negative test indicates that their baby will not have brain damage.

   b. follow-up testing should be done during one of the early clinic visits.

   c. the test must be done before the infant nurses or has any formula.

   d. a special diet begun when the infant takes solid food will prevent disability.

7. Erythromycin ointment is instilled in a newborn's eyes to prevent infection by

   a. rubella.

   b. syphilis.

   c. gonorrhea.

   d. herpes.

8. The nurse gives a postpartum woman a rubella immunization. Which is the most important client teaching related to this immunization?

   a. Let someone else care for your baby if you have a rash.

   b. Use a reliable birth control method for three months.

   c. Avoid prolonged exposure to the sun for two to three weeks.

   d. Increase your fluid intake if you develop a fever.

9. The drug given to the newborn to prevent hemorrhage is

   a. erythromycin.

   b. naloxone.

   c. vitamin K.

   d. triple dye.

10. Blood for glucose testing should be obtained from the

    a. scalp vein using a "butterfly" needle.

    b. umbilical cord stump.

    c. fetal surface of the placenta.

    d. lateral surface of the heel.

11. What should the mother be taught about perineal cleansing?

    a. Do perineal cleansing only after bowel movements.

    b. Cleanse from back to front with soft wipes.

    c. Direct the flow of fluid from the front to the back.

    d. Do not use disposable wipes on the perineal area.

12. Colostrum's greatest benefit to the infant is prevention of

    a. constipation.

    b. weight loss.

    c. hemorrhage.

    d. infection.

Student Name Shirley Williams S.P.N.

13. The let-down reflex is stimulated by
    a. massage of the uterus.
    b. suckling of the baby.
    c. increased fluid intake.
    d. breast engorgement.

14. What should the nursing mother be taught about breast care?
    a. Use plain water to wash the breasts.
    b. Absorb excess milk with plastic-backed pads.
    c. Do not wear a bra the first few days after birth.
    d. Begin with the same breast at each feeding.

15. Choose the best position for the newborn after feeding.
    a. on his/her back
    b. on his/her abdomen
    c. upper body elevated
    d. side-lying

16. At her two-week postpartum check-up, the woman's uterus should be
    a. two fingerwidths above the umbilicus.
    b. two fingerwidths below the umbilicus.
    c. just above the symphysis pubis.
    d. no longer palpable through the abdomen.

17. Diuresis in the early postpartum period indicates
    a. urinary tract infection.
    b. retention of body fluids.
    c. excretion of excess fluid.
    d. edema near the urinary meatus.

18. The earliest time when sexual intercourse can usually be resumed after birth is
    a. at two weeks postpartum.
    b. when the episiotomy heals.
    c. when lochia serosa is present.
    d. after the six-week check.

19. The most appropriate parent teaching about care of the infant's umbilical area is to
    a. keep a small dressing over the cord.
    b. allow air to circulate near the area.
    c. report drying or crusting to the doctor.
    d. position the infant on his/her abdomen.

20. The most appropriate way to identify mother and infant when reuniting them is to
    a. check the identification band numbers of each.
    b. ask the mother to clearly state her name.
    c. examine the mother's fingerprint and infant's footprints.
    d. verify that the names on the infant's crib card and band are identical.

21. Which is the best nursing measure to increase the woman's perineal comfort during the first hour after vaginal birth with a midline episiotomy?
    a. Help her take a warm sitz bath.
    b. Give her an oral analgesic drug.
    c. Apply topical anesthetic ointment.
    d. Place an ice pack on the area.

22. A mother phones the postpartum unit three days after birth. She says her baby cannot suck well on her nipples because her breasts are full and engorged. What should the nurse recommend?

    a. Apply ice packs just before allowing the infant to nurse.

    b. Feed formula for the next two feedings to reduce pain and congestion.

    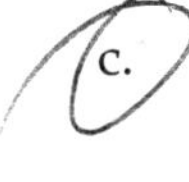

    c. Massage the breasts and express a small amount of milk before nursing.

    d. Reduce daily liquid intake to one quart for a few days.

23. The nurse notes that a new mother has several bottles of partly consumed formula on her overbed table. Choose the most appropriate nursing action.

    a. Recommend that she prepare bottles that contain only what the baby is likely to drink.

    b. Inform her that the bottles cannot be used because they have not been refrigerated.

    c. Tell her she may combine the leftover formula for the baby's next feeding.

    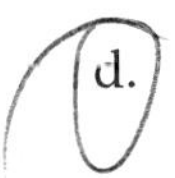

    d. Check the room for other partially-used bottles, then throw all of them in the trash.

24. Which lochia characteristic should the nurse teach the woman to report?

    a. change from red to pink-brown to white

    b. cessation of flow by four weeks postpartum

    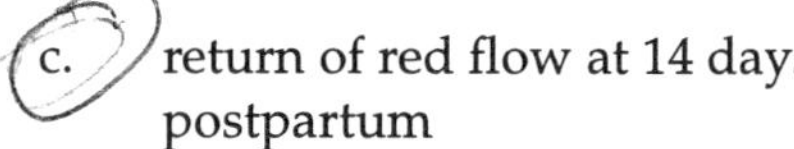

    c. return of red flow at 14 days postpartum

    d. presence of a menstrual-like odor

25. The nurse should interpret a new mother's passive behavior during the first few hours after birth as

    a. a normal characteristic of the taking-in phase.

    b. a likely sign of impaired parent-infant bonding.

    c. evidence of ambivalence about the baby.

    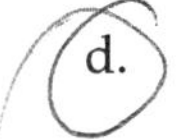

    d. reluctance to assume the mothering role.

Student Name ______________________________

chapter **10**

Nursing Care of Women with Complications Following Birth

LEARNING ACTIVITIES

1. Match the terms in the left column with their definitions on the right (a–j).

J curettage	a. infection of the uterine lining
A metritis	b. infection of the breast
I hematoma	c. lodging of a blood clot in a blood vessel of the lung
D Homan's sign	d. calf pain when the foot is dorsiflexed
E hypovolemic shock	e. inadequate amount of blood to maintain normal circulation
G mania	f. psychiatric disorder characterized by impairment of reality
B mastitis	g. hyperactive, excitable, euphoric behavior
F psychosis	h. delayed return of the uterus to its nonpregnant state
C pulmonary embolism	i. collection of blood within tissues
H subinvolution	j. scraping or vacuuming the inner surface of the uterus

2. Postpartum hemorrhage is blood loss that exceeds 500 ml after vaginal birth or 1000 ml after cesarean birth.

3. Early postpartum hemorrhage occurs within 24 hours of birth; late postpartum hemorrhage occurs later than 24 hours after birth until 6 weeks after birth.

4. Describe the following five changes that occur in hypovolemic shock and indicate the change or changes that usually occur early.

   a. Heart rate Tachycardia (rapid heart rate) is usually the 1st sign of inadequate blood volume

   b. Respiratory rate increase the

   c. Blood pressure ______

   d. Skin and mucous membranes ______

   e. Mental state ______

5. Why does a poorly contracted uterus lead to hemorrhage?

6. What is the connection between the infant suckling at the breast and limitation of postpartum bleeding?

7. Describe typical differences in bleeding and uterine fundus characteristics between hemorrhage caused by uterine atony and that caused by a birth canal laceration.

   a. Bleeding

      Uterine atony ______

      Laceration ______

Student Name ____________________

b. Uterine fundus

Uterine atony ____________________

____

____

____

Laceration ____________________

____

____

8. Describe the following typical manifestations of a birth canal hematoma.

a. Visual appearance ____________________

____

b. Character of pain or pressure ____________________

____

____

c. Signs of blood loss ____________________

____

9. How does manual removal of the placenta differ from the usual method of separation?

____

____

____

10. Distinguish between the characteristics of a superficial vein thrombosis (SVT) and a deep vein thrombosis (DVT).

a. SVT ____________________

____

b. DVT ____________________

____

11. The greatest risk of deep vein thrombosis is that it may result in ____________________.

12. Postpartum infection is generally characterized by a temperature of ________________ after the first ________ hours after birth, occurring on at least ____________ days of the first ______________ days after birth.

13. List the localized signs and symptoms of infection.

    ____

14. List the generalized (systemic) signs and symptoms of infection.

    ____

15. Why may the white blood cell (leukocyte) count be unreliable to diagnose infection after birth? ____

    ____

16. Why are postpartum infections in the reproductive tract likely to spread?

    ____

    ____

17. What nutritional teaching about infections is important?

    ____

    ____

    ____

18. Distinguish between *cystitis* and *pyelonephritis* in terms of the following characteristics.

    a. Fever ____

    ____

    b. Discomfort ____

    ____

    ____

    c. Other characteristics ____

    ____

    ____

19. Describe the following nursing measures to promote recovery from urinary tract infection and prevent future ones.

    a. Fluid intake ____

    ____

Student Name ______________________________

b. Beneficial foods ______________________________

____

20. Which two factors increase the likelihood that mastitis will develop?

a. ______________________________

b. ______________________________

21. What is the role of heat application in the care of a woman with mastitis?

a. ______________________________

b. ______________________________

c. ______________________________

22. Describe two characteristics of subinvolution of the uterus.

a. ______________________________

____

b. ______________________________

____

23. Describe the basic difference between postpartum "blues" and postpartum depression.

a. Postpartum "blues" ______________________________

____

b. Postpartum depression ______________________________

____

____

THINKING CRITICALLY

1. How can the nurse's teaching about breastfeeding reduce the likelihood that a woman will develop mastitis?

CASE STUDY

1. Carmen Esparza had a cesarean delivery after a long labor. Her daughter weighed 10 pounds at birth and is apparently healthy. Carmen's blood loss during her surgery was 1,200 ml. She has an indwelling catheter, and the bag contains 550 ml of light-yellow urine when she is admitted to the recovery room. The dressing over her vertical incision is clean, dry, and intact. Carmen is awake and has not yet regained sensation from her epidural anesthetic, although she can move her legs.
   a. Identify the priority nursing diagnosis for Carmen during her recovery period. What interventions are appropriate for this nursing diagnosis?
   b. If Carmen's urine output decreases, what should the nurse suspect?
   c. What complications are more likely to develop later in the postpartum period?

OTHER LEARNING ACTIVITIES

1. Look at the graphic charts of several postpartum women. What is the pattern of their temperature and pulse rates after birth?
2. Study the routine postpartum teaching given to all women before discharge. For each sign or symptom that a woman should report, identify the complications related to that sign or symptom.
3. Determine if your clinical facility provides written postpartum self-care instructions in languages other than English. If not, what provisions does the staff make for non-English–speaking clients?

REVIEW QUESTIONS

1. A woman had a forceps-assisted birth two hours ago. Baseline vital signs were temperature 37.1°C (98.8°F), pulse 78, respirations 20, blood pressure 118/70. Which of the following assessments suggests possible development of hypovolemic shock?
   a. firm fundus, slightly right of midline
   b. pulse 100, respirations 22
   c. respirations 22, blood pressure 112/76
   d. moderate lochia rubra with small clots

2. A woman had a 16-hour labor that ended with the cesarean birth of a 4,313 g (9.5 lb) infant. Her membranes were ruptured for 24 hours and oxytocin augmentation of labor was necessary. She has an IV infusion and indwelling catheter. Which complication should the nurse be most observant for during her immediate recovery room period?
   a. uterine atony
   b. endometritis
   c. uterine subinvolution
   d. urinary tract infection

Student Name ____________________

3. If the nurse finds that a new mother's uterus is soft, the appropriate initial action is to
   a. insert an indwelling catheter.
   b. massage the uterus until firm.
   c. check the woman's vital signs.
   d. increase the rate of the IV fluid.

4. An hour after vaginal birth, the nurse notes that a woman has a flat purple area, about 2 cm by 3 cm, on her perineum. Which is the most appropriate nursing action at this time?
   a. Assist her to take a warm sitz bath.
   b. Apply pressure with a tightly applied pad.
   c. Place a chemical cold pack on the area.
   d. Notify the physician of the observation.

5. When teaching a woman following vaginal birth 24 hours ago, the nurse should tell her to report
   a. pink vaginal drainage followed by red drainage.
   b. menstrual-like odor of vaginal discharge.
   c. uterine cramping when the infant nurses.
   d. excretion of large quantities of dilute urine.

6. Choose the most appropriate intervention to prevent deep vein thrombosis in a woman who is one day postcesarean birth.
   a. Encourage her to walk several times each day.
   b. Provide her with increased fluids that she enjoys.
   c. Take her temperature to identify an elevation.
   d. Instruct her to stay in bed most of the day.

7. Choose the finding that suggests infection after birth.
   a. poorly relieved perineal pain four hours postpartum
   b. oral temperature of 37.7°C (100°F) 18 hours postpartum
   c. white blood cell count of 21,000/dl at one day postpartum
   d. persistent and severe cramping three days postpartum

8. The best position for the woman who has postpartum metritis is
   a. semi-sitting.
   b. side-lying.
   c. supine.
   d. prone.

9. Which nursing assessment suggests that a postpartum woman has cystitis?
   a. frequent passage of small amounts of urine
   b. high fever with occasional chilling
   c. fever accompanied by nausea and vomiting
   d. voiding large amounts of dilute urine

10. Which nurse's teaching is appropriate for the new mother who has cystitis?
    a. Eat several servings of whole grains and meats each day.
    b. Remain in bed except for going to the bathroom.
    c. Drink about three liters of noncaffeinated beverages daily.
    d. Take a stool softener to reduce added pain of constipation.

11. A woman is eight hours postpartum after a spontaneous vaginal birth. Her admission hemoglobin was 10 g/dl, and her estimated blood loss during the birth was 750 ml. She asks the nurse if she can walk to the bathroom. The best nursing response is to

    a. remind her that she should catch her urine in a "hat" to be measured.

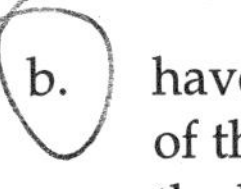

    b. have her sit briefly on the side of the bed before helping her to the bathroom.

    c. encourage her to urinate every two hours to decrease the risk of excess bleeding.

    d. tell her to return to bed promptly after she finishes using the bathroom.

12. Which nursing assessment suggests infection of a episiotomy?

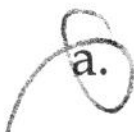

    a. temperature of 38°C (100.4°F) 12 hours after birth

    b. purplish discoloration of the perineum and labia

    c. edema of the labia minora, labia majora, and perineum

    d. redness of the perineum with separation of the suture line

13. A woman has postpartum uterine atony with hemorrhage. After it is controlled, the physician orders an indwelling Foley catheter mainly because it

    a. allows better estimation of the woman's blood volume.

    b. identifies bloody urine that suggests bladder trauma.

    c. limits the need for the woman to ambulate to the bathroom.

    d. applies constant pressure against the bleeding uterus.

14. A woman who is three days postpartum comes to the emergency clinic because she is having pain and burning discomfort when she urinates. She denies that she has had any fever. The nurse should expect an initial order for

    a. bladder analgesics.

    b. intravenous antibiotics.

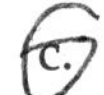

    c. complete blood count.

    d. catheterized urine specimen.

15. A woman is five days postpartum and breastfeeding. She telephones the nurse at the clinic and says that her breasts feel very heavy and one of them is tender. She says the infant nurses "fair." The nurse should tell the woman that

    a. her symptoms should go away when the infant begins nursing better.

    b. breastfeeding should be stopped until the pain goes away.

    c. a cold pack between feedings should reduce the pain.

    d. she should come to the clinic for evaluation of her symptoms.

16. Methylergonovine (Methergine) should be avoided if the woman has

    a. uterine atony.

    b. retained placenta.

    c. hypertension.

    d. endometritis.

17. Which of these postpartum women is at greatest risk for bleeding from a vaginal wall laceration?

    a. She had a forceps-assisted vaginal birth.

    b. She delivered an 8 lb (3,632 g) infant.

    c. She has a history of uterine atony.

    d. Oxytocin (Pitocin) was used to induce labor.

Student Name ______________________

18. Choose the foods that are highest in iron.
    a. citrus fruits, apricots, tomatoes
    b. sweet and white potatoes, corn, dried beans
    c. whole grains, dark green leafy vegetables
    d. milk, cheeses, legumes

19. A woman comes to the clinic for her six-week postpartum check after having her first baby. She says to the nurse, "I don't know what's wrong with me. I'm exhausted all the time and yet I can't seem to sleep when I have the chance." The nurse should
    a. reassure her that the demands of being a mother can seem overwhelming, especially with the first baby.
    b. ask her if her partner, family members, or friends can help her with care of the baby and her home so she can rest.
    c. explain that women lose more blood at birth than they expect, and a slight anemia often leads to these symptoms.
    d. find a quiet place to talk with her about her feelings related to her new role as a mother.

20. Postpartum bipolar disorder is characterized by
    a. periods of let-down feelings but with general enjoyment of life.
    b. impaired reality characterized by euphoria alternating with depression.
    c. alternate periods of overeating and disinterest in food and drink.
    d. prolonged feelings of worthless-ness or guilt.

chapter **11**

Nurse's Role in Women's Health Care

LEARNING ACTIVITIES

1. Match the terms in the left column with their definitions on the right (a–j).

_____ basal temperature
_____ climacteric
_____ dyspareunia
_____ endometriosis
_____ infertility
_____ laminaria
_____ menopause
_____ osteoporosis
_____ spinnbarkeit
_____ varicocele

a. painful sexual intercourse
b. presence of tissue resembling uterine lining outside the uterus
c. cones of a substance that absorbs water to begin cervical dilation
d. stretching of the cervical mucus at ovulation
e. body temperature at rest, taken before any activity
f. inability to conceive when desired
g. enlarged vein in the scrotum
h. cessation of menstruation
i. period of time surrounding the cessation of menstruation
j. loss of bone mass leading to bone fragility

2. a. The best time to perform breast self-examination is ______________________________ or ______________________________.

   b. Professional breast examination should be done ____________ for all women over the age of _________.

   c. 1998 recommendations of the American Cancer Society for mammography is that the procedure be done for all women aged _________ at ____________ intervals.

Student Name ______________________________

3. List the two preparations needed for a Pap test.

   a. ______________________________

   b. ______________________________

4. a. The Pap test is recommended at ______________ intervals for all women age __________ or older.

   b. Under what conditions can a Pap test be done less frequently?

   ____

   ____

5. Define each term that relates to menstrual disorders.

   a. Amenorrhea ______________________________

   ____

   b. Primary amenorrhea ______________________________

   ____

   c. Secondary amenorrhea ______________________________

   ____

   d. Metrorrhagia ______________________________

   ____

   e. Menorrhagia ______________________________

   ____

   f. Mittelschmerz ______________________________

   ____

   g. Dysmenorrhea ______________________________

   ____

6. How can body weight relate to amenorrhea?

   ____

   ____

7. List each criterion required to diagnose premenstrual syndrome (PMS).

   a. ______________________________

   ____

   b. ______________________________

   ____

   c. ______________________________

   ____

   d. ______________________________

   ____

8. Explain each type of induced abortion.

   a. Therapeutic ______________________________

   ____

   b. Elective ______________________________

   ____

9. Describe important teaching related to toxic shock syndrome in each area listed.

   a. Hand washing

   ____

   ____

   b. Use of tampons

   ____

   ____

   c. Use of cervical cap or diaphragm for contraception

   ____

   ____

10. The sexually transmitted disease (STD) characterized by intense itching, inflammation of the vulva, and burning on urination is ____________________.

Student Name ______________________________

11. How can infections of *Chlamydia* or gonorrhea result in infertility or an ectopic tubal pregnancy?

____

____

____

12. The STD that has three possible stages is ____________.

13. Infections of ____________ can re-emerge later in outbreaks that are also infectious.

14. Most oral contraceptives contain ____________ and ____________, while some contain only ____________.

15. What is the significance of the *ACHES* acronym in relation to oral contraceptives? What does each letter stand for?

____

____

____

____

____

____

16. A major side effect of the Norplant contraceptive implant is ____________. It should be removed in ____________ years.

17. Depo-Provera provides ______ months of contraception. It is given by the ____________ route within ______ days of the menstrual period. Why is it given at this time?

18. Three common side effects of Depo-Provera are:

    a. ______________________________

    b. ______________________________

    c. ______________________________

19. What is the major difference between the ParaGard and the Progestasert intrauterine devices?

____

____

____

20. List two times when the diaphragm must be refitted.

    a. ______________________________

    b. ______________________________

21. Describe appropriate teaching about condom use in each area listed.

    a. Lubrication ______________________________

    ____

    b. Breakage or dislodgment during use ______________________________

    ____

    c. Expiration date ______________________________

    ____

    d. Removal ______________________________

    ____

22. List and describe three methods that can be used for natural family planning.

    a. ______________________________

    ____

    b. ______________________________

    ____

    c. ______________________________

    ____

23. Why must another form of contraception be used for about one month following vasectomy?

    ____

    ____

24. Explain why each of these methods is not reliable for contraception.

    a. Withdrawal ______________________________

    ____

    b. Douching ______________________________

    ____

Student Name ______________________________

c. Breastfeeding ______________________________

____

25. Describe the psychologic reactions a couple may have to infertility.

____

____

____

____

____

26. Describe similarities and differences among *in vitro* fertilization (IVF), gamete intrafallopian transfer (GIFT), and tubal embryo transfer (TET).

____

____

____

____

____

27. State what occurs in these hormones during the climacteric.

a. Follicle-stimulating hormone ______________________________

____

b. Estrogen ______________________________

____

c. Progesterone ______________________________

____

28. Describe the possible sensations a woman feels when she has a "hot flash."

____

____

____

29. Describe changes in these structures that occurs with loss of estrogen.

    a. Uterus and ovaries ______________________________

    ____

    b. Vagina ______________________________

    ____

    c. Pelvic musculature ______________________________

    ____

    d. Bones ______________________________

    ____

    e. Heart and blood vessels ______________________________

    ____

30. Explain the advantages of hormone replacement therapy.

    ____

    ____

    ____

31. Describe each variation of vaginal wall prolapse.

    a. Cystocele ______________________________

    ____

    b. Enterocele ______________________________

    ____

    c. Rectocele ______________________________

    ____

32. What is/are the usual treatment(s) for uterine leiomyomas?

    ____

    ____

THINKING CRITICALLY

1. When in your orthopedic experience, note how many women are affected with hip fractures compared to the number of men affected. Do you notice other signs of osteoporosis in these clients?

Student Name ______________________________

OTHER LEARNING ACTIVITIES

1. Interview nurses at a clinic about their experience caring for clients with STDs. Which diseases are most prevalent?

2. Under supervision, teach a woman to perform a breast self-examination.

REVIEW QUESTIONS

1. The nurse is teaching a woman, age 25, about breast self-examination (BSE). The correct teaching is that BSE

   a. detects malignancy more often than professional examinations.

   b. allows her to delay the need for mammography until she is 50 years old.

   c. helps her learn what are normal characteristics for her own breasts.

   d. is more accurate than a yearly mammogram.

2. Choose the correct teaching about breast self-examination technique.

   a. Use the palms of the hand to press the breast tissue firmly against the ribs.

   b. Palpate each breast systematically, using the pads of the fingers.

   c. Palpate the underarm area only if the breasts are very large and sagging.

   d. Squeeze the breast tissue between the thumb and index finger.

3. Choose the correct teaching for relief of premenstrual syndrome symptoms.

   a. Eat hard candies several times each day to keep the blood sugar high.

   b. Limit intake of water to six glasses to reduce fluid retention and edema.

   c. Plan the most stressful activities during the last half of the menstrual cycle.

   d. Do aerobic exercise several times each week.

4. When teaching about the use of tampons, the nurse should emphasize replacing them at least every four hours to prevent

   a. pelvic inflammatory disease.

   b. vasomotor symptoms.

   c. STDs.

   d. toxic shock syndrome.

5. A friend asks you what she can do because she is troubled by repeated "yeast" infections. As a nurse, your best advice to her is to

   a. keep over-the-counter medications on hand so she can begin treatment immediately.

   b. see her physician or nurse-practitioner if she has another infection to identify possible causes.

   c. increase her intake of fluids to include at least eight glasses of water each day.

   d. avoid sexual intercourse for one month to see if that reduces the infections.

6. The long-term risk of an infection with the human papilloma virus is for
   a. cervical cancer.
   b. ectopic pregnancy.
   c. endometriosis.
   d. nerve damage.

7. Besides abstinence, the best way to prevent sexually transmitted infection with the human immunodeficiency virus is
   a. douching within 30 minutes of sexual intercourse.
   b. avoiding intercourse during midcycle.
   c. use of a condom for all episodes of sexual intercourse.
   d. taking prophylactic antibiotics after unprotected intercourse.

8. Choose the most appropriate teaching for the woman who is prescribed multiphasic oral contraceptive pills.
   a. Take one pill each day for three weeks; omit pills for seven days; repeat.
   b. Reduce cigarette smoking to no more than 10 per day.
   c. Limit intake of foods that are high in iron or calcium.
   d. Take the pills at the same time of day and in order.

9. A woman should not take the oral contraceptive if she
   a. has multiple sexual partners.
   b. smokes more than 15 cigarettes daily.
   c. is younger than 18 years old.
   d. is formula-feeding her new baby.

10. A woman has been taking oral contraceptives for four months. She is concerned because her periods are much lighter than before she started the pills. How should the nurse counsel this woman?
    a. "You will probably have to discontinue the pill unless your periods become more like they were previously."
    b. "We can switch you to a barrier contraceptive; your periods should return to normal in just a few months."
    c. "Lighter periods are expected when you are on the pill but you should tell us if they stop entirely."
    d. "Stop taking the pills immediately. We want to do a pregnancy test before you resume them."

11. Choose the correct client teaching about the IUD.
    a. "You should not use this contraception if you smoke or are over 35."
    b. "Check for the strings weekly for the first four weeks, then monthly."
    c. "Do not use tampons when you have your menstrual period."
    d. "Use another contraception for the first month after insertion."

12. Other than abstinence, the contraceptive method that provides the best protection against STDs is the
    a. female condom.
    b. hormone implant.
    c. intrauterine device.
    d. contraceptive sponge.

Student Name ______________________________

13. When teaching a woman the cervical mucus method to identify ovulation, the nurse teaches her that the character of the mucus near ovulation is
    a. slippery and stretchy.
    b. yellowish with a distinct odor.
    c. cloudy and sticky.
    d. thick, sticky, and clear.

14. Appropriate client teaching following vasectomy is to
    a. apply heat to the operative area for 20 minutes at a time.
    b. abstain from intercourse for at least six weeks after the surgery.
    c. limit frequency of sexual intercourse for the first month.
    d. place an ice pack on the operative area to reduce discomfort.

15. A friend tells you that she is "having periods again." She thought she had her last menstrual period two years ago. As a nurse, you should advise her that she
    a. is probably having reactivation of estrogens that are causing the bleeding.
    b. should see a physician promptly because this is not an expected occurrence.
    c. may be ovulating again and should use a contraceptive if she does not want to become pregnant.
    d. probably has an infection of her vagina or cervix that should be treated to prevent further infection.

16. "Hot flashes" are probably caused by
    a. anxiety about growing older and one's mortality.
    b. shifts in a woman's fluid and electrolyte balance.
    c. instability of the blood pressure.
    d. fluctuating levels of estrogen and progesterone.

17. Choose the correct client teaching about the drug alendronate (Fosamax).
    a. Take food or milk within 30 minutes of the medication.
    b. Wash the nose out with saline 30 minutes after using the spray.
    c. Do not lie down for at least 30 minutes after taking the drug.
    d. Take calcium supplements at the same time as the medication.

18. Stress incontinence is best described as loss of urine
    a. during activities such as laughing or coughing.
    b. when in an anxiety-provoking situation.
    c. occurring with pressure on the suprapubic area.
    d. during sexual intercourse.

19. What is the usual diagnostic procedure when an ovarian cyst is suspected?
    a. transvaginal ultrasound examination
    b. bimanual pelvic examination
    c. laparotomy with biopsy
    d. magnetic resonance image

20. A nursing measure that can improve stress incontinence is to

    a. teach the woman to limit fluid intake to eight glasses of water each day.

    b. advise her to increase her fiber intake with raw vegetables and fruits and whole grains.

    c. encourage weight-bearing exercise at least three times each week.

    d. explain how and when to perform the Kegel exercise.

Student Name ______________________________

chapter **12**

The Term Newborn

LEARNING ACTIVITIES

1. Match the terms in the left column with their definitions on the right (a–h).

_____ acrocyanosis
_____ circumcision
_____ cryptorchidism
_____ Epstein's pearls
_____ fontanelle
_____ hypospadias
_____ milia
_____ Mongolian spots

a. urethral opening on underside of penis
b. bluish hands or feet
c. small white bumps, usually on the nose or chin
d. removal of the foreskin of the penis
e. blue areas, usually on the sacrum or buttocks
f. failure of the testes to descend into the scrotum
g. soft area at the intersection of skull bones
h. white dots on the hard palate

2. Describe each reflex and state the age at which it is expected to disappear.

a. Moro ______________________________

____

b. Rooting ______________________________

____

c. Tonic neck ______________________________

____

3. Normal newborn head circumference is from ______________ inches to ________ inches, or from ____________ cm to ____________ cm.

4. List two functions of an infant's fontanelles.

   a. ____

   ____

   b. ____

   ____

5. Describe the following characteristics of the anterior fontanelle.

   a. Shape ____

   b. Location (bones) ____

   c. Time of closure ____

6. Describe the following characteristics of the posterior fontanelle.

   a. Shape ____

   b. Location (bones) ____

   c. Time of closure ____

7. Describe the three steps for using a bulb suction to remove excess secretions.

   a. ____

   b. ____

   c. ____

8. Explain the two types of heart murmurs that can be heard in newborns. Indicate which may cause problems.

   a. Functional ____

   ____

   b. Organic ____

   ____

9. a. What is a common route of taking a newborn's temperature initially?

   ____

   b. Subsequent temperatures are taken by what route?

   ____

Student Name ____________________

c. What is the correct technique for taking the temperature by each method?

____

____

10. Give the following newborn vital signs that the nurse should promptly report.

a. Temperature higher than ______°F or lower than ______°F. (Celsius equivalents are higher than ______°C or lower than ______°C.)

b. Pulse higher than ______ bpm or lower than ______ bpm.

c. Respirations higher than ______ breaths/minute or lower than ______ breaths/minute

11. Give the average newborn measurements.

a. Length ______ to ______ inches (______ to ______ cm)

b. Weight ______ to ______ pounds (______ to ______ g)

12. Describe the following normal musculoskeletal assessments for a newborn, including any possible deviations from normal.

a. Movements ____________________

____

b. Eyes ____________________

____

____

c. Tremors ____________________

____

d. Muscle tone ____________________

____

13. Describe the following characteristics and functions of a newborn infant's kidneys.

a. Blood flow ____________________

____

b. Reabsorption functions ____________________

____

c. Concentration of urine ____

____

d. Capacity to handle fluid imbalances ____

____

14. List the pros and cons of circumcision.

a. Pros ____

____

b. Cons

____

____

15. Circumcision is usually performed on the __________ day after birth in Jewish families.

16. Describe postcircumcision nursing care in terms of the following.

a. Comforting ____

____

b. Bleeding ____

____

c. Urination ____

____

17. Explain the normal occurrences that cause physiologic jaundice.

____

____

____

____

____

____

18. Physiologic jaundice appears at about __________ days after birth and lasts for about __________ days.

Student Name ______________________________

19. Describe the following typical stools in the newborn, including the time they appear, if applicable.

    a. Meconium ______________________________

    ____

    b. Transitional stool ______________________________

    ____

    c. Stool of breastfed baby ______________________________

    ____

    d. Stool of bottle-fed baby ______________________________

    ____

20. Describe three types of abnormal stools in the newborn.

    a. ______________________________

    b. ______________________________

    c. ______________________________

21. Describe stools in constipation.

    ____

    ____

22. The newborn's stomach has a capacity of about __________ ml and empties in about ____________ hours.

23. Why is it important to prevent infection in a newborn and why may it be difficult to recognize?

    ____

    ____

CASE STUDY

1. Sandra and Jim Black, a couple in their mid-20s, have a new baby son named Justin who is 12 hours old and is breastfeeding. Sandra expects to go home 36 hours after birth. Justin will be circumcised (Plastibell) before discharge. Sandra and Jim have no nearby relatives and are the first couple in their circle of friends to have a baby. They have read books on baby care, but are concerned about actually caring for their baby's needs. Sandra and Jim say they need to know "everything." For each area listed, explain what content you will teach them. How can you include "hands-on" care by the parents so they will feel more secure? How will you incorporate information they may have read in books? You are encouraged to incorporate any of your facility's teaching materials as you complete this case study.

   a. positioning

   b. safety

   c. using bulb syringe

   d. maintaining body temperature

2. Because Justin will be discharged shortly after being circumcised, what should you teach the parents about care and observation for complications? How can they comfort him?

OTHER LEARNING ACTIVITIES

1. Assist with admitting newborns after birth. Administer prophylactic eye care and vitamin K injections. What initial and ongoing cord care does your facility use? Does your facility offer the first hepatitis-B immunization with newborn care? Do parents sign a consent form for any of these procedures? Which one(s)?

2. Observe newborns in the nursery for characteristics that were listed in the textbook. Distinguish between normal characteristics and those that may indicate a problem. What action is taken for deviations from normal?

3. Observe a circumcision. What type of circumcision is most common in your hospital? Observe newborns after circumcision for bleeding and urination.

4. Does your hospital have an infant care teaching plan for new parents? If so, what does the plan include? Observe how different staff nurses incorporate parent teaching into their care of mothers and babies. How have short stays influenced parent teaching?

Student Name ______________________________

REVIEW QUESTIONS

1. Which reflex shows the baby reaction to sudden movement by drawing up the legs and folding the arms across the chest?

   a. dancing

   b. Moro

   c. rooting

   d. grasp

2. Which newborn reflex is used when teaching breastfeeding?

   a. Moro

   b. gag

   c. tonic neck

   d. rooting

3. In the birthing room, a first-time father asks the nurse why the baby's head is "long and pointy." The nurse should respond

   a. "The head changes shape so it can pass through the mother's pelvis during birth."

   b. "Fluid builds up within the head before and during birth; it will go away in a few days."

   c. "Labor causes slight bleeding into the space between the skull bones and their covering."

   d. "We will notify the pediatrician, who will probably order an MRI of the baby's head."

4. Visually, babies prefer

   a. geometric objects.

   b. soft, blending colors.

   c. the human face.

   d. nonmoving objects.

5. The correct way to suction a baby's mouth with a bulb syringe is to

   a. depress the bulb, place the tip in the side of the mouth, then release the bulb.

   b. place the tip in the side of the mouth, depress the bulb, then release the bulb.

   c. depress the bulb, place the tip in the center of the mouth, then release the bulb.

   d. place the tip in the center of the mouth, depress the bulb, then release the bulb.

6. An infant's initial rectal temperature is 96.6°F (35.8°C). Choose the most appropriate nursing response for this assessment.

   a. Chart the temperature and continue other observations.

   b. Recheck the temperature in 30 minutes to verify it.

   c. Remove blankets and sources of heat from the baby.

   d. Wrap the baby in warm blankets and report the temperature.

7. One hour after circumcision, the nurse notes a small amount of blood oozing from the area. Which is the appropriate initial nursing response to this observation?

   a. Continue observing for increased bleeding.

   b. Apply pressure with a gauze pad and gloved fingers.

   c. Call the physician who performed the procedure.

   d. Wrap petroleum jelly (Vaseline) gauze around the penis.

8. A new mother asks why her two-day-old baby's skin is yellow. Which is the best nursing response to explain the cause of this skin color?
   a. Small blood vessels are broken during labor, releasing waste products into the blood.
   b. The baby's digestive tract is immature and cannot excrete bilirubin.
   c. Skin color changes slightly during the first few weeks until the permanent color is evident.
   d. Excess blood cells are being broken down rapidly because the baby is now breathing air.

9. New parents should be taught to clean their baby's ears by
   a. moistening a cotton-tipped applicator with water and rotating it in the ear canal.
   b. gently instilling a small amount of warm water into the ear with a bulb syringe.
   c. applying baby oil to a rolled piece of cotton and inserting it into the ear.
   d. wiping the outside with cotton that is moistened with water.

10. When a small area of a term baby's abdominal skin is pinched gently, the skin remains distorted. This suggests
    a. dehydration.
    b. overhydration.
    c. normal edema.
    d. immature turgor.

11. What should the parents be taught about bathing the newborn before the cord site heals?
    a. Give the baby a tub bath.
    b. A sponge bath is advised.
    c. Use an oil-based cleanser.
    d. Avoid bathing the baby.

12. The primary complication for a newborn who has a skin abrasion at birth is
    a. bleeding.
    b. hypothermia.
    c. jaundice.
    d. infection.

13. A newborn has blood drawn for laboratory studies. The mother is concerned because the baby is crying loudly. The best response of the nurse is
    a. "That's the only way the baby can communicate with us."
    b. "Hold the baby close and comfort him by gentle rocking."
    c. "Babies cannot feel pain because they are immature."
    d. "The baby will only cry for a few minutes at most."

14. How should the nurse respond to acrocyanosis in a 12-hour-old infant?
    a. Administer oxygen through an infant-sized mask.
    b. Apply heat with an incubator or radiant warmer.
    c. Assess the pulse and respirations for abnormal rates.
    d. Continue routine newborn nursing observations.

15. Which is an abnormal assessment for a term newborn at three days of age?
    a. Twelve percent of birth weight is lost.
    b. The apical pulse is 130/bpm.
    c. Bluish areas appear on the sacral area.
    d. Tiny white spots occur on the nose.

Student Name ____________________

16. A new mother asks why her baby shakes when he cries. Choose the best nursing response.

    a. "We will ask the baby's doctor about this."

    b. "The baby is probably just easily upset."

    c. "An infant's muscles are too weak to move steadily."

    d. "This is a normal infant behavior during crying."

17. The first meconium stool is usually passed no later than ______ hours after birth?

    a. 6

    b. 12

    c. 24

    d. 36

18. A new mother is concerned because her three-day-old daughter has a slightly blood-tinged vaginal mucus discharge. How should the nurse respond to this mother's concern?

    a. "The baby could have a minor abnormality in her vagina."

    b. "Has there been any kind of injury to this area?"

    c. "Effects of your pregnancy hormones cause this response."

    d. "This should be reported to the doctor right away."

19. The nurse should teach parents to avoid using baby powder because it

    a. irritates the respiratory tract.

    b. may cause allergies in the newborn.

    c. is difficult to remove during a bath.

    d. dries the skin of the axillae and groin.

20. An infant looks at her mother and remains quiet when the mother sings to her in soft, high-pitched tones. This is an example of

    a. signs of possible impaired hearing.

    b. the quiet alert state of reactivity.

    c. sensory overload due to sound stimulus.

    d. limited ability to respond to adults.

chapter **13**

Preterm and Postterm Newborns

LEARNING ACTIVITIES

1. Match the terms in the left column with their definitions on the right (a–g).

_____ apnea
_____ atelectasis
_____ Dubowitz
_____ gestational age
_____ hyperalimentation
_____ kernicterus
_____ surfactant

a. provision of full nutrition by the parenteral (IV) route
b. length of time spent in the uterus
c. cessation of breathing for 20 seconds or more
d. lung secretion that facilitates oxygen exchange
e. nervous system damage caused by high levels of bilirubin in the blood
f. unexpanded lung tissue
g. method of estimating newborn maturity by physical characteristics

2. a. A preterm infant's gestational age is less than ____________ weeks.

   b. A term infant's gestational age is __________ to __________ weeks.

   c. A postterm infant's gestational age is greater than _____________ weeks.

3. Describe the following typical physical characteristics of a preterm infant's appearance.

   a. Skin ____

   b. Superficial veins ____

   c. Subcutaneous fat ____

   d. Lanugo ____

Student Name ______________________________

e. Vernix caseosa ______________________________

f. Sole creases ______________________________

g. Abdomen ______________________________

h. Nails ______________________________

i. Genitalia ______________________________

4. Respiratory distress syndrome (RDS) is associated with an inadequate quantity of ______________________ in the lungs.

5. If preterm birth appears inevitable, the physician may order what drug to be given to the mother to accelerate production of fetal lung surfactant?

   ____

6. List two signs that may accompany apnea.

   a. ______________________________

   b. ______________________________

7. Bradycardia in the infant is a pulse rate lower than __________ bpm.

8. List seven factors that make the preterm infant especially vulnerable to loss of body heat.

   a. ______________________________

   b. ______________________________

   c. ______________________________

   d. ______________________________

   e. ______________________________

   f. ______________________________

   g. ______________________________

9. A preterm baby is prone to hypoglycemia because stores glycogen and fat are __________ and because the demand for glucose is __________.

10. *Hypoglycemia* is defined as a plasma level of glucose lower than ______________ mg/dl.

11. Preterm newborns are prone to bleeding because they have a low level of ______________________________ and because their capillaries are ______________________.

12. Describe five factors that impair the preterm infant's nutritional function.

    a. ______________________________

    b. ______________________________

    c. ______________________________

    d. ______________________________

    e. ______________________________

13. Necrotizing enterocolitis (NEC) is characterized by bowel ______________ ______________. It may result in ______________.

14. The upper limit of bilirubin concentration in physiologic jaundice is ________ mg/dl in the term infant and ________ mg/dl in the preterm infant.

15. The ideal milk for the preterm infant is ______________ milk.

16. List three methods by which the preterm infant can receive nourishment.

    a. ______________________________

    b. ______________________________

    c. ______________________________

17. A good position for the preterm infant after feeding is on the ______________ side with the head slightly ______________.

18. Describe the following typical physical characteristics of the postterm newborn.

    a. General body appearance ______________

    b. Presence of lanugo ______________

    c. Presence of vernix caseosa ______________

    d. Skin appearance ______________

THINKING CRITICALLY

1. A friend had her baby at 32 weeks gestation six months ago. She confides that she is afraid her baby is not normal because he does not do the same things her first baby (born full-term) did at six months old. What can you tell your friend to reassure her?

Student Name ______________________________

OTHER LEARNING ACTIVITIES

1. Observe newborns of different gestational ages in your clinical facility. Identify differences in these characteristics. Determine whether the mother's "due date" correlates with the physical characteristics you see.
   a. head and body hair
   b. body posture and muscle tone
   c. stiffness of ear cartilage
   d. amount of breast tissue
   e. appearance of genitalia
   f. number and depth of sole creases
2. Observe different methods of feeding preterm infants. What precautions are taken to ensure that the baby is receiving adequate nutrition without overload?
3. If your facility does not routinely care for sick newborns, does it have arrangements with a larger hospital to transport these babies to a special care nursery? What is involved in transporting a sick baby? When do most newborns return to the original facility?
4. How does your facility foster parent-infant attachment when an infant is sick or preterm? Is kangaroo care used?
5. What treatment is used for jaundice that exceeds safe limits in your facility? Look up the protocols for nursing care that accompany this treatment.

REVIEW QUESTIONS

1. Which of the following physical characteristics is typical of a preterm infant?
   a. large amount of subcutaneous fat
   b. abundant amount of lanugo
   c. labia majora cover labia minora
   d. nails extend to end of fingers
2. Gestational age is best described in terms of the
   a. weight of the infant at birth.
   b. adequacy of placental blood supply.
   c. maturation of the infant after birth.
   d. duration of residence *in utero*.
3. A preterm infant is subject to hypothermia because the
   a. brain heat regulating center is absent.
   b. insulating fat is excessive.
   c. sweat glands are overactive.
   d. body surface area is large.
4. The nurse should interpret a plasma glucose level of 28 mg/dl in the preterm infant as
   a. minimally normal.
   b. hypoglycemic.
   c. hyperglycemic.
   d. predictive of brain injury.

5. The nurse must handle the preterm infant gently because capillaries are

   a. not developed in all areas of the brain.

   b. more likely to develop microscopic clots.

   c. sensitive to high levels of clotting factors.

   d. fragile and prone to bleed spontaneously.

6. The advantage of radiant heaters in the care of preterm infants is that they

   a. cannot cause excessive body temperature.

   b. maintain warmth with easy caregiver access.

   c. reduce drying and cracking of the skin.

   d. improve balance of fluids and electrolytes.

7. The ideal feeding for most preterm newborns is

   a. glucose water.

   b. breast milk.

   c. special formula.

   d. hyperalimentation.

8. When doing the admission assessment on an infant, the nurse notes that the infant has peeling skin and a long, thin appearance. What should the nurse check in the mother's chart related to the infant's appearance?

   a. medications received during labor

   b. possible blood incompatibility

   c. duration of second-stage labor

   d. estimated date of delivery

9. A mother gives birth to a preterm infant at 30 weeks gestation. When visiting the baby in the intensive care unit, she seems interested in the baby, but sits and watches everything the nurse does for her baby. Which is the most appropriate nursing intervention to promote mother-infant attachment?

   a. Invite her to provide simple care to her infant.

   b. Reassure her that she can hold the baby soon.

   c. Stress the importance of frequent visits to the nursery.

   d. Demonstrate the skills she will need for home care.

10. Which nursing assessment most suggests respiratory distress syndrome?

   a. respiratory rate 35 breaths/minute, hypoglycemia, red skin color

   b. grunting, rapid respirations, nasal flaring

   c. protruding abdomen, irregular respirations

   d. mottled skin color, hypocalcemia, nasal flaring

11. The alarm on an apnea monitor for a preterm infant sounds. The infant is asleep and the skin color is pink. The most appropriate initial nursing response is to

   a. contact the physician for orders.

   b. gently rub the infant's back.

   c. give oxygen with an Ambu bag.

   d. suction the infant with a bulb syringe.

Student Name ____________________

12. A key nursing intervention to prevent retinopathy of prematurity is to
    a. provide early glucose water feedings.
    b. disturb the infant as little as possible.
    c. eliminate potential sources of infection.
    d. closely monitor arterial blood gases.

13. Most problems of the postterm infant are the result of
    a. decreased functioning of the placenta.
    b. reduced blood clotting factors.
    c. increased susceptibility to infection.
    d. increased subcutaneous fat deposits.

14. The best way to determine an infant's gestational age is to
    a. assess body length and rate of weight gain.
    b. observe physical and neurologic characteristics.
    c. identify signs associated with respiratory distress.
    d. check the mother's chart for estimated date of delivery.

chapter **14**

The Newborn with a Congenital Malformation

LEARNING ACTIVITIES

1. Match the terms in the left column with their definitions on the right (a–g).

_____ habilitation

_____ kernicterus

_____ macrosomia

_____ Ortolani's sign

_____ Pavlik's harness

_____ simian crease

_____ transillumination

a. inspection of a cavity or organ by passing a light through its walls

b. suggestive of developmental hip dysplasia

c. teaching a skill to a child who is handicapped from birth

d. maintains hip abduction in the treatment of developmental hip dysplasia

e. single transverse line across the palm

f. brain damage due to accumulation of bilirubin in the brain

g. large fetal or newborn body size

2. List five types of problems that the neonate may have.

a. ______________________________

b. ______________________________

c. ______________________________

d. ______________________________

e. ______________________________

Student Name ______________________________

3. Give the two classifications of hydrocephalus and describe each.

   a. ______________________________

   ____

   b. ______________________________

   ____

4. List two possible complications of shunts for treatment of hydrocephalus.

   a. ______________________________

   b. ______________________________

5. Why is it essential to frequently change the position of a child who has hydrocephalus?

   ____

   ____

6. Describe other nursing observations and care that are important for the child with hydrocephalus.

   ____

   ____

   ____

   ____

7. List signs of the two primary complications that may occur after shunt placement for hydrocephalus.

   a. Infection of the shunt ______________________________

   ____

   b. Increased intracranial pressure ______________________________

   ____

8. A ______________________________ is a form of spina bifida in which portions of the membranes and cerebrospinal fluid are contained in a cystic mass.

9. A ______________________________ is a form of spina bifida that consists of protrusion of a sac-like cyst containing meninges, spinal fluid, and a portion of the spinal cord with its nerves.

10. What is the current recommendation for all women related to prevention of neural tube defects such as meningomyelocele?

____

____

11. Describe nursing observations and care for the newborn with spina bifida in each of these areas.

    a. Care of the sac ______________________________

    ____

    b. Extremities ______________________________

    ____

    c. Head ______________________________

    ____

    d. Bowel and bladder function ______________________________

    ____

12. What options are there for positioning the child with a myelocele or meningomyelocele?

____

____

13. Describe postoperative nursing care for the child with a cleft lip repair.

    a. ____

    ____

    b. ____

    ____

    c. ____

    ____

    d. ____

    ____

    e. ____

    ____

    f. ____

    ____

Student Name ______________________________

14. List four ways of treating clubfoot.

    a. ______________________________

    b. ______________________________

    c. ______________________________

    d. ______________________________

15. Describe nursing care of the child who has a cast on both legs.

____

____

16. List four signs of developmental hip dysplasia.

    a. ______________________________

    ____

    b. ______________________________

    ____

    c. ______________________________

    ____

    d. ______________________________

    ____

17. What procedure should be used to turn a child in a body cast?

____

____

____

____

____

____

18. Explain how and when infants are screened for PKU.

____

____

____

19. Describe each of these inborn errors of metabolism and their treatment.

    a. Maple syrup urine disease ______________________________

    ____

    b. Galactosemia ______________________________

    ____

20. Describe characteristics that may be seen in a child with Down syndrome.

    ____

    ____

21. Parents of children born with Down syndrome have special needs. Give three examples of how the nurse can meet these needs.

    a. ______________________________

    ____

    b. ______________________________

    ____

    c. ______________________________

    ____

22. Describe pathophysiology of erythroblastosis fetalis.

    ____

    ____

23. Erythroblastosis fetalis can be prevented by the administration of ______________________________.

24. Describe care of the child receiving phototherapy in an incubator in each of the following areas.

    a. Eye protection ______________________________

    ____

    b. Genital protection ______________________________

    ____

    c. Potential dehydration ______________________________

    ____

Student Name ____

25. Intracranial hemorrhage can result from ________________ or ____________________________________.

26. List signs that you might observe in an infant with an intracranial hemorrhage.

____

____

____

____

27. What are two possible permanent effects of an intracranial hemorrhage?

    a. ____

    b. ____

28. It is essential to monitor ________________ closely immediately after an infant of a diabetic mother is born. Why? ____

____

____

What is the normal level? ____

THINKING CRITICALLY

1. If you have a pediatric client with Down syndrome, compare the development of gross and fine motor abilities of that child with those of a child of the same approximate age who does not have Down syndrome. (Also see Chapter 15 in your text for information on normal growth and development.) This exercise might also be done if you are acquainted with a family who has a child with Down syndrome. Has the child with Down syndrome had any of the associated problems, such as respiratory infections, ear infections, or heart defects?

CASE STUDIES

1. Timmy is a newborn who has a meningomyelocele. Timmy's legs are paralyzed and he is dribbling urine and stool.
    a. Identify four nursing concerns for the nurse caring for Timmy.
    b. What can the nurse tell Timmy's mother about the dribbling of urine and oozing of stool as it relates to skin care and future control of these functions?
    c. How should the nurse involve the parents in Timmy's care in the newborn nursery?
    d. What related problems should the nurse observe for in Timmy?

2. Four-month-old Dianna is brought to the hospital by her mother because she had a seizure this morning. The admission physical exam shows an irritable, thin, lethargic child who the mother says has been vomiting the small amount of formula she would eat. Her height and weight measurements are below the third percentile and her head circumference is in the 90th percentile. Dianna has not had any health care since her birth in a distant city. The admitting diagnosis is suspected hydrocephalus.

   a. Is Dianna exhibiting any signs of increased intracranial pressure? List observations that would support your conclusion.

   b. What diagnostic test will be done to confirm this diagnosis?

   c. What nursing measures should the nurse take to promote skin integrity?

   d. How should the nurse position Dianna during and after feedings?

4. Jonathan, a three-week-old infant, is admitted for repair of a bilateral cleft lip. He also has a cleft palate which will be repaired later.

   a. Describe methods the nurse will use to feed Jonathan.

   b. What is the purpose of the Logan bow and the use of restraints postoperatively?

   c. What precaution should be used related to Jonathan's arm restraints?

   d. What nursing interventions are appropriate for each of these concerns?

      i. Postoperative nutrition

      ii. Protection of the operative area

      iii. Facilitating parent-infant attachment

OTHER LEARNING ACTIVITIES

1. While in the clinical area, care for a child who has Down syndrome.

2. Observe the repair of a cleft lip or cleft palate.

3. Care for an infant receiving phototherapy.

4. Feed an infant with a cleft lip or cleft palate.

Student Name ____

REVIEW QUESTIONS

1. A classic sign of hydrocephalus would be an increase in
   a. activity.
   b. amount of hair.
   c. milk intake.
   d. head size.

2. Expected treatment for hydrocephalus is
   a. placement of a shunt.
   b. incision and draining.
   c. oral diuretics.
   d. intravenous analgesics.

3. Symptoms of increased intracranial pressure include
   a. increased blood pressure and pulse.
   b. decreased blood pressure and pulse.
   c. decreased blood pressure and increased pulse.
   d. increased blood pressure and decreased pulse.

4. The usual position of a newborn with a meningomyelocele is
   a. side-lying with a pillow between the legs.
   b. prone with a pad between the legs.
   c. supine with the legs elevated.
   d. supine with the legs widely abducted.

5. Which of the following nursing measures is appropriate for an two-week-old infant who has had a cleft lip repair?
   a. position on the abdomen or side
   b. prevent crying as much as possible
   c. provide a premature-sized pacifier
   d. limit visitors to immediate family

6. Appropriate nursing care for a nine-month-old infant who has cleft palate repair includes
   a. padded side rails.
   b. elbow restraints.
   c. a Logan bow.
   d. continuous sedation.

7. Appropriate care related to a wet cast for correction of clubfoot in the newborn includes
   a. keeping the infant snugly wrapped until the cast is dry to prevent hypothermia.
   b. putting a small amount of powder into the dry cast to reduce skin irritation.
   c. position in a slight feet-dependent position to promote circulation.
   d. leaving the toes uncovered to assess color and pulses.

8. A child with developmental hip dysplasia is likely to exhibit ____________________ of the leg on the affected side.
   a. limitation of abduction
   b. full leg abduction
   c. limitation of adduction
   d. limited thigh flexion

9. A sign of intracranial hemorrhage in an infant is
   a. depressed fontanelle.
   b. shrill cry.
   c. constant sucking.
   d. constricted pupils.

10. The child with PKU must be on a diet that is
    a. low in Lofenalac.
    b. high in soluble fiber.
    c. low in phenylalanine.
    d. fluid restricted.

11. Early identification of many inborn errors of metabolism is required to prevent
    a. depletion of specific amino acids.
    b. excess accumulation of some amino acids.
    c. damage to the genitourinary system.
    d. restriction of normal growth.

12. Appropriate nursing care for parents immediately after the birth of a baby who has characteristics typical of Down syndrome should include
    a. reassuring them that any future babies are unlikely to have Down syndrome.
    b. keeping the infant in the nursery until a definitive diagnosis is made.
    c. spending time with them and facilitating the grieving process.
    d. teaching them about special nutritional care the baby will need.

13. Parent-infant bonding can be enhanced in an infant with an unrepaired meningomyelocele by
    a. encouraging the parents to talk to and touch the baby.
    b. having the parents change the baby's diaper.
    c. encouraging the parents to hold the baby closely.
    d. helping the parents bathe the baby each day.

14. The mother of a two-week-old infant who is going to have a cleft lip repair asks if she will be able to hold her baby after surgery. The nurse should reply
    a. "Not until the sutures are removed."
    b. "It would be very unlikely."
    c. "Yes, you should try to keep your baby happy."
    d. "Not until the baby is taking formula well."

15. Infants should be screened for PKU at age
    a. 8 hours.
    b. 16 hours.
    c. 24 hours.
    d. 72 hours.

16. Treatment of a child with a clubfoot should begin
    a. shortly after birth.
    b. when he begins to stand.
    c. before he walks.
    d. when he begins walking.

17. One method of feeding the one-year-old infant who is postoperative following a cleft palate repair is with a
    a. straw.
    b. cup.
    c. bottle.
    d. soft tongue depressor.

Student Name ______________________________

18. Expected advice for the woman with PKU who is considering pregnancy is to eat a daily diet that
    a. is rich in high-fiber foods.
    b. contains adequate dairy products.
    c. provides added amounts of leucine.
    d. has low quantities of phenylalanine.

19. The infant with Down syndrome is at increased risk for developing
    a. urinary tract infections.
    b. respiratory infections.
    c. kidney infections.
    d. meningitis.

20. The nurse should particularly observe the newborn of a diabetic mother for what complication immediately after birth?
    a. intracranial hemorrhage
    b. reduced level of consciousness
    c. excessive urination
    d. low blood glucose levels

21. Why might an infant of a diabetic mother be small for gestational age (SGA)?
    a. The placenta did not receive adequate perfusion during pregnancy.
    b. The fetus had episodes of hypoglycemia when the mother took insulin.
    c. The fetal pancreas cannot manufacture insulin if the mother takes insulin.
    d. The mother's diabetes causes small areas of bleeding in the placenta.

chapter **15**

An Overview of Growth, Development, and Nutrition

LEARNING ACTIVITIES

1. Match the terms in the left column with their definitions on the right (a–g).

_____ cephalocaudal
_____ development
_____ growth
_____ maturation
_____ parallel play
_____ physiologic anemia
_____ proximodistal

a. progressive increase in physical size
b. progressive increase in body function
c. total way a person grows and develops, dictated by inheritance
d. head-to-toe developmental pattern
e. central-to-peripheral developmental pattern
f. fall in the hemoglobin at three to four months as the fetal hemoglobin disappears
g. activity alongside another child or children

2. List the age range (in months or years) of each of the following stages.

a. Fetus ______________________________

b. Newborn ______________________________

c. Infant ______________________________

d. Toddler ______________________________

e. Preschool child ______________________________

f. School-age child ______________________________

g. Adolescent ______________________________

Student Name ______________________________

3. Give a specific example of each type of developmental pattern.

   a. Cephalocaudal ______________________________

   ____

   b. Proximodistal ______________________________

   ____

4. What are the two most rapid periods of growth after birth?

   a. ______________________________

   b. ______________________________

5. Birth weight usually ______________________ by six months of age and ______________________ by one year.

6. How does the percentage of body fluid change as the infant matures to adulthood? Why is it important for the nurse to know this?

   ____

   ____

   ____

   ____

7. Why would a burn chart for calculating percentage of body surface area injured be inappropriate for the child with burns?

   ____

   ____

   ____

   ____

8. Why are ear infections more common in young children?

   ____

   ____

   ____

   ____

9. List the components of the *family APGAR*.

   A ____

   P ____

   G ____

   A ____

   R ____

10. Give an example of each of Piaget's stages of cognitive development. For best learning, give examples other than those listed in your text.

    a. Sensorimotor __________________________________

    b. Preoperational __________________________________

    c. Concrete operations ______________________________

    d. Formal operations ______________________________

11. How can parents' knowledge of growth and development help prevent accidents in children?

12. A mother is concerned that her child is not "keeping up" with her friend's child. If the child's development is within ranges for his age, what would you say to the mother?

13. Why might a child who eats a vegetarian diet be anemic?

Student Name ______________________________

14. "Solids" should be introduced to children at what age? ______________

15. Children should continue on breast milk or iron-fortified formula until what age? ______________ What is the earliest age that a child should begin whole milk? ______________

16. Why should fat and cholesterol not be limited in infants and young children?

____

____

____

17. One guideline for determining the appropriate amount of food to feed to children is ______________ tablespoon(s) of food for each year of age.

18. What are the causes of bottle mouth caries? ______________________________

____

What is the prevention measure for them? ______________________________

____

19. What is the first-aid measure for traumatic loss of a permanent tooth?

____

____

____

____

20. Care of a child's teeth should include which four components?

a. ______________________________

b. ______________________________

c. ______________________________

d. ______________________________

21. What is the chief difference between the play of several toddlers (ages one to two years) and play of several preschoolers (ages three to five years)?

____

____

____

THINKING CRITICALLY

1. Observe a child in the clinical area. Based on the assessment, determine which of Erikson's stages of development the child is attempting to accomplish. Give at least three examples of observed behavior that support your choice.

2. Using the information provided in Table 15-6 in the textbook and the food pyramid, develop a meal plan for a nine-year-old child using foods unique to that child's ethnic background.

OTHER LEARNING ACTIVITIES

1. a. Plot the height and weight of the following children on the growth chart (Figure 15-4 in the textbook).

Age	Height	Weight
4 years	38 in.	40 lb
8 years	52 in.	60 lb
12 years	58 in.	65 lb

   b. What percentile does each of the above children fall into?

   c. Which child would need further evaluation of his growth?

2. Plan a menu for a four-year-old hospitalized child on a general diet. Include serving size and how the food is best served in your plan.

3. While in the clinical setting, instruct a mother about her infant's dietary needs.

REVIEW QUESTIONS

1. A child must be able to sit before he can walk. This is an example of which directional pattern?
   a. cephalocaudal
   b. proportional
   c. proximodistal
   d. linear

2. One of the most accurate indicators of biologic age is
   a. height.
   b. weight.
   c. bone growth.
   d. teeth eruption.

3. According to Piaget, the 7- to 11-year-old child is at which of the following stages of cognitive development?
   a. sensorimotor
   b. formal operations
   c. concrete operations
   d. proportional

4. Dental caries are prevented through the administration of oral
   a. iodine.
   b. fluoride.
   c. sodium.
   d. iron.

Student Name ____________________

5. Most children are able to feed themselves using a spoon by age
   a. 12 months.
   b. 15 months.
   c. 2 years.
   d. 3 years.

6. The theorist known for his work on moral development is
   a. Freud.
   b. Kohlberg.
   c. Sullivan.
   d. Piaget.

7. A current comic strip depicts a family in which parents, children, and the children's grandfather live together. This is an example of
   a. nuclear family.
   b. alternate family.
   c. extended family.
   d. reconstituted family.

8. Blood cholesterol levels below which level are considered acceptable in children and adolescents?
   a. < 170 mg/dl
   b. < 180 mg/dl
   c. < 200 mg/dl
   d. < 220 mg/dl

9. What age should all children begin brushing their teeth?
   a. three years
   b. four years
   c. five years
   d. six years

10. A hospitalized preschool child picks at her food and is generally a "finicky" eater. The nurse should
    a. insist that the child eat.
    b. remove the tray without comment.
    c. ask another nurse to try to get her to eat.
    d. encourage the parents to be present at mealtimes.

11. Which of the following statements would most likely have the most positive outcome when counseling adolescents on nutrition?
    a. "If you don't eat properly now, you may have heart trouble when you get older."
    b. "You will get run down and sick if you don't eat properly."
    c. "Shiny hair and good muscles are linked to good nutrition."
    d. "If you eat nutritiously, you won't have acne."

12. When assessing a child's weight and height at a preschool clinic visit, the nurse plots his weight on the growth chart. The nurse notes that the weight is in the 95th percentile for the child's height. Based on this assessment, the nurse should
    a. encourage the mother to feed the child two additional snacks each day.
    b. recommend an intake of at least four glasses of whole milk each day.
    c. question the mother and child about the type and quantity of foods eaten in a typical day.
    d. look for other signs of poor nutrition, such as a distended abdomen or circles under the eyes.

13. A practice that should be discouraged is

    a. allowing a two-year-old child to brush his teeth.

    b. feeding a six-month-old infant iron-fortified cereal.

    c. putting a one-year-old infant to bed with a bottle of formula.

    d. rocking a nine-month-old infant before bedtime.

14. Solids are generally introduced to children at age

    a. 4 months.

    b. 6 months.

    c. 8 months.

    d. 10 months.

15. Formula-fed infants should continue on iron-fortified formula until

    a. the introduction of solid foods.

    b. they drink from a cup.

    c. 6 months of age.

    d. 12 months of age.

Student Name ____________________

chapter **16**

The Infant

LEARNING ACTIVITIES

1. Match the terms in the left column with their definitions on the right (a–g).

_____ crawling

_____ creeping

_____ extrusion reflex

_____ grasp reflex

_____ object permanence

_____ parachute reflex

_____ pincer grasp

a. closure of the hand when the palm is stimulated

b. automatically pushing food out of the mouth

c. extension of both arms when thrust downward in the prone position

d. forward self-propulsion with lower body contacting floor

e. forward self-propulsion with trunk above and parallel to floor

f. accurate opposition of index finger and thumb of same hand

g. infant can remember that an object exists, even if it is out of sight

2. Sucking is an important activity for the young infant because it provides

a. ____________________

b. ____________________

3. How can the nurse help meet the infant's sucking needs during the following?

a. Oral feedings ____________________

____

____

b. Intravenous fluid therapy ____

____

____

4. The primary need for normal personality development during infancy is to acquire a sense of ________________________.

5. Appropriate types and amounts of sensory stimulation help develop the infant's

a. ____

b. ____

6. State the age when the following key events in an infant's growth and development are likely to occur.

a. _______ months: elevates upper body with arms

b. _______ months: sits from a standing position

c. _______ months: imitates facial expressions

d. _______ months: two lower central incisors; begins to crawl; transfers objects from one hand to the other

e. _______ months: birth weight tripled; may walk

f. _______ months: sits alone; pincer grasp

g. _______ months: walks holding furniture; deliberately throws objects on floor

h. _______ months: turns from back to side

i. _______ months: can place a toy in pan

j. _______ months: grasps objects; puts everything in mouth

7. What are three points that the nurse should emphasize to the parents to promote childhood immunization?

a. ____

b. ____

c. ____

8. Give examples of routine examinations at well-baby health checks.

____

____

____

Student Name ______________________________

9. List four factors that influence nutritional needs during infancy.

   a. ______________________________

   b. ______________________________

   c. ______________________________

   d. ______________________________

10. List health benefits of breastfeeding for the infant.

   a. ______________________________

   b. ______________________________

   c. ______________________________

   d. ______________________________

11. How can you teach a new mother that her baby has had sufficient breast milk at a feeding?

   ____

   ____

   ____

12. What food should be avoided for two years to prevent botulism in infants and young children? ______________________________

13. Current recommendations are that solid foods be introduced to the infant's diet at about ____________ months. Why?

   ____

   ____

14. What is the first solid food usually introduced to the infant? ____________ Why?

   ____

   ____

15. Why should the nurse recommend that parents introduce only one new food to the infant at a time?

   ____

   ____

16. List six foods that are usually delayed until the baby is one year old.

    a. ______________________________

    b. ______________________________

    c. ______________________________

    d. ______________________________

    e. ______________________________

    f. ______________________________

17. Why should parents not limit fat in the diets of children and infants younger than two years?

    ____

    ____

THINKING CRITICALLY

1. A mother is concerned because her four-month-old baby does not seem to be developing as quickly as her sister's baby, who is about the same age. What should the nurse tell this mother about infant development?

2. When caring for an infant on pediatrics, talk with parents about their baby's personality. Is their infant irritable, crying at handling or other stimulation, or calm when handled or meeting new people? How does the infant's behavior affect the parents or other family members?

3. Ask several parents how they cared for their colicky infant. How long did the infant have colic? How did it affect the family?

CASE STUDIES

1. You are teaching the parents of Sarah, a healthy newborn who is being discharged with her mother. Formulate appropriate parent teaching in each of the following areas.

    a. immunizations (first year)

    b. sleeping all night

    c. colic

2. Danny, six months old, is visiting the clinic for his immunizations and check-up. His parents will begin feeding "solid" foods now. What should you teach his parents in each of the following areas?

    a. order of introducing solid foods

    b. foods to avoid and how long to avoid them

    c. avoiding infections acquired from foods

Student Name ____________________

OTHER LEARNING ACTIVITIES

1. Determine the most common infant formulas recommended by physicians or pediatric nurse-practitioners in your clinical facility. What special infant formulas are readily available in the newborn nursery or the pediatric unit and when are these prescribed?

2. As you care for infants in maternity and pediatric nursing clinical experiences, assess for reflexes listed in Chapter 16 of the textbook.

REVIEW QUESTIONS

1. The primary personality development during the first year is to acquire
   a. independence.
   b. prehension.
   c. trust.
   d. consistency.

2. The primary use of growth and development guidelines is to
   a. help parents anticipate their child's changing needs.
   b. compare children of similar ages with each other.
   c. predict general intelligence and school performance.
   d. identify the child who is mentally retarded.

3. Which is the correct developmental milestone to be expected for the child's age?
   a. Passes a toy from one hand to the other at three months.
   b. Uses the root reflex to seek the nipple at five months.
   c. Sits without support at six months.
   d. Pulls to standing position at 10 months.

4. The mother of a two-month-old is bringing her to the office for a routine check-up and immunizations. She says the baby cries quite a bit but she just lets her cry so she won't become "spoiled." As a nurse, the best response is to
   a. tell the mother she should also lower the lights and play soft music or other "white noise."
   b. explain that babies this young cannot be spoiled, then give her some ideas to help soothe the baby.
   c. encourage the mother to continue helping her baby become more independent.
   d. reassure the mother that she probably just has an irritable baby, but that this phase will not continue for long.

5. The best position for an infant to sleep in is
   a. prone.
   b. sitting in an infant seat.
   c. on the parents' bed.
   d. side-lying or supine.

6. During infancy, which organ system is most critical for continued growth and development?
   a. gastrointestinal
   b. central nervous
   c. cardiopulmonary
   d. musculoskeletal

7. If a parent wants to microwave formula before feeding, the nurse should

   a. explain that microwaving can overheat the formula and cause severe burns.

   b. tell the parent that cold formula preserves the nutrients better than heating it.

   c. advise the parent to wait until the infant takes at least eight ounces of formula at each feeding.

   d. give guidelines for microwaving and caution the parent to test the temperature of the formula before feeding.

8. The primary focus of routine infant health care is to

   a. prevent disease.

   b. accelerate development.

   c. reduce allergies.

   d. assess growth rate.

9. A mother wants to know if she can keep leftover strained baby food. Choose the best nursing response.

   a. "Discard any food that the baby doesn't eat after it is opened."

   b. "Refrigerate the leftover food within two hours after it is opened."

   c. "When the baby has eaten all she wants from the jar, promptly refrigerate the remainder."

   d. "Remove the amount of food you think the baby will eat from the jar and refrigerate the rest."

10. A formula often prescribed for the infant who cannot tolerate cow's milk formulas is based on

    a. goat's milk.

    b. soybeans.

    c. rice.

    d. artificial protein.

11. New foods should be introduced into the infant's diet no faster than every _________ days.

    a. 1–2

    b. 3

    c. 4–7

    d. 14

12. Social development that is common for the two-month-old infant is

    a. responsive smiling.

    b. laughing aloud.

    c. recognizing his/her own name.

    d. anxiety around strangers.

13. When bringing her nine-month-old baby in for a check-up, a new mother asks if she can feed the baby puréed fish since this is a low-fat food that is a staple in the family's diet. The best response of the nurse is

    a. "It is never too early to begin a heart-healthy diet."

    b. "Fish protein is one of the best quality proteins available."

    c. "You can try, but many infants dislike the taste of fish."

    d. "Fish is more likely than other meats to cause allergies."

14. Crawling often begins when the infant is ___________ months old.

    a. 4

    b. 7

    c. 9

    d. 12

Student Name ______________________________

15. Which is the most important teaching about use of the microwave for heating infant food?
    a. Use less time than would be needed for larger pieces of food.
    b. Rotate the food two or more times while warming it.
    c. Avoid heating foods that are higher in fat, such as meat.
    d. Test the temperature of any warmed food on the inner wrist.

16. A fruit that should be delayed until after the infant's first birthday is
    a. strawberries.
    b. applesauce.
    c. apricots.
    d. pears.

17. Safety considerations when choosing toys for a five month old should assume that all of them will go into her
    a. tub.
    b. food.
    c. mouth.
    d. bed.

18. Minor head lag when pulling a one-month-old infant to the sitting position
    a. is an expected finding.
    b. demonstrates prematurity.
    c. identifies poor nutrition.
    d. suggests developmental delay.

19. By the age of one year, an infant's weight should be
    a. twice the birth weight.
    b. three times the birth weight.
    c. about 16 pounds.
    d. about 25 pounds.

20. The nurse can reassure parents that their infant's colic will probably not last beyond the age of
    a. one month.
    b. three months.
    c. six months.
    d. nine months.

21. The baby can usually be offered finger foods such as zwieback crackers beginning at about age
    a. three months.
    b. five months.
    c. seven months.
    d. nine months.

22. A good initial method to deal with a nine-month-old infant who is attracted to a dangerous situation is to
    a. shout a quick, loud "No!".
    b. take his favorite toys away.
    c. spank him with one light blow.
    d. distract him from the situation.

chapter 17

The Toddler

LEARNING ACTIVITIES

1. Match the terms in the left column with their definitions on the right (a–f).

_____ ambivalence	a. independent play in company of other children
_____ autonomy	b. playing with other children
_____ cooperative play	c. consistent, recurring pattern of behavior
_____ egocentric thinking	d. having conflicting feelings and reactions at the same time
_____ parallel play	e. thinking in reference to oneself
_____ ritualism	f. self-control

2. Give the age when the toddler is expected to achieve each developmental milestone.

   a. _________ months: can undress self, throws ball

   b. _________ months: imitates adults' activities, holds spoon

   c. _________ months: begins to share, uses tricycle

3. According to Erickson, the major developmental task for the toddler is to acquire _________________ and overcome __________________ and ___________________________.

4. What are the expected average vital signs for a two-year-old?

   a. Pulse: _____________ to ____________ bpm

   b. Respirations: _____________ to ____________ breaths/minute

   c. Blood pressure: _________ mmHg

Student Name ______________________________

5. List two self-consoling behaviors that toddlers exhibit.

   a. ______________________________

   b. ______________________________

6. List four indications of readiness for toilet training.

   a. ______________________________

   b. ______________________________

   c. ______________________________

   d. ______________________________

7. Excessive milk intake that reduces the amount of solid foods may lead to a deficiency of what element? ______________________

   This can result in what condition? ______________________

8. Two characteristics of the toddler's eating habits are that the appetite ______________________ and food preferences are ______________________.

9. A good guide for approximate serving size of solid foods for the toddler is ______________ per ______________.

10. When talking to the toddler, the adult should be at the child's ______________________.

11. Bladder training is more likely to succeed if the toddler stays dry for about __________ hours.

12. Why is it important to teach the toddler generally recognized words to signal a need to use the bathroom?

    ____

    ____

    ____

    ____

13. When using "time out" with children, parents can determine the time by limiting it to ______ minute(s) per year of age.

14. List three interventions that can assist parents with the toddler during bedtime.

    a. ______________________________

    b. ______________________________

    c. ______________________________

15. List two methods of preventing injuries in children that are mandated by law.

    a. ______________________________

    b. ______________________________

16. ______________________ are the leading cause of childhood death.

THINKING CRITICALLY

1. How can you help parents deal with the fears of their toddler? Why is it important for adults to control their own fears around a toddler?

2. How can you use assessment of a child's growth and development to provide better care for him/her when he/she is hospitalized?

3. How can parents' knowledge of a child's expected growth and development help protect the child from injury?

4. How is full myelination of the spinal cord related to success of toilet training?

CASE STUDY

1. Tommy is a two-year-old whose mother is frustrated because of his temper tantrums when he is disciplined. What can you teach Tommy's mother about discipline at his age? How can knowledge of normal growth and development be used to teach his mother about setting limits?

OTHER LEARNING ACTIVITIES

1. Use growth charts to determine if the physical growth of hospitalized children is normal.

2. Discuss daycare with classmates who are parents. Are they satisfied with the care their children receive? Have they had problems with daycare?

REVIEW QUESTIONS

1. Compared to growth during infancy, a toddler's growth rate is

    a. faster.

    b. slower.

    c. inconsistent.

    d. unchanged.

2. When helping a toddler choose clothing for the day, the best approach is to

    a. ask him what he wants to wear.

    b. ask which of two appropriate outfits he prefers.

    c. select the best outfit for the weather.

    d. remove all inappropriate clothing from his closet.

Student Name ______________________________

3. The position that best facilitates adult-child conversation is
   a. at the child's eye level.
   b. above the child's eye level.
   c. standing while the child sits.
   d. both seated at a small table.

4. When teaching parents of the toddler about eating, the nurse should stress that the toddler
   a. prefers a variety of foods mixed on the plate.
   b. must usually be coaxed to eat adequately.
   c. eats one food for a while, then rejects it.
   d. usually enjoys regular addition of new foods.

5. The mother of a two-year-old asks the nurse whether she should begin toilet training now. The most appropriate nursing response is
   a. "Your child is too young for toilet training to be successful."
   b. "About how much time elapses between changes of wet diapers?"
   c. "How important is this skill to you and your family?"
   d. "It should be fairly easy to toilet train your child now."

6. Automobile child restraint devices should be used when the child
   a. begins sitting in the rear seat.
   b. crawls about in the car.
   c. resists activity restraints.
   d. travels anywhere in the car.

7. Select the toy that is *inappropriate* for a toddler.
   a. balloon
   b. blocks
   c. sand box
   d. pull toy

8. Which is the best description of a toddler's language ability?
   a. Describing actions precedes naming objects.
   b. Words are used for their shock effect on adults.
   c. Talking to the child may delay speech development.
   d. Understanding is more developed than verbalization.

9. Choose the best description of physical changes during the toddler years.
   a. Head growth slows and chest growth continues.
   b. Muscle size and strength remain steady.
   c. Body temperature regulation is erratic.
   d. Ability to fight infections is less than during infancy.

10. The nurse can best help reduce accidental injuries to toddlers by

    a. limiting the number of toys available to them at one time.

    b. teaching parents about expected changes in their abilities.

    c. providing written information about common child hazards.

    d. using restraints whenever the child is uncooperative.

11. A mother is concerned because her 14-month-old child has "quit talking." Choose the most appropriate initial nursing response.

    a. "Your child may be concentrating on walking right now."

    b. "Children prefer to listen after they begin talking."

    c. "Your child might have a slight hearing loss."

    d. "Talking isn't very purposeful at this age anyway."

12. When assessing a two-year-old child hospitalized for minor day surgery, the nurse should expect that the pulse rate will be about ___________ bpm.

    a. 60–80

    b. 70-110

    c. 125–135

    d. 120–140

13. When buying shoes for their toddler, parents should choose those that provide

    a. a firm, straight sole to facilitate walking.

    b. a strong arch to prevent "fallen" arches.

    c. protection from objects that might injure the feet.

    d. adequate movement of the heel within the shoe.

14. While caring for an eight-month-old infant, you observe that although the child cries, he does not coo or babble. You know that

    a. infants usually begin to make sounds at about 10 months.

    b. by six months, the infant should be cooing and babbling.

    c. the important milestone is that the infant is crying.

    d. the doctor would have said something if this behavior is abnormal.

15. A mother asks you what she should do about her two-year-old child's temper tantrums. The best response is

    a. "He must not be getting enough attention."

    b. "If you let him get away with temper tantrums now, he will really be a problem when he gets older."

    c. "Have you tried rewarding his good behavior?"

    d. "You might try putting him in his room for 30 minutes."

Student Name ______________________________

chapter **18**

The Preschool Child

LEARNING ACTIVITIES

1. Match the terms in the left column with their definitions on the right (a–f).

_____ animism

_____ artificialism

_____ centering

_____ diurnal

_____ egocentrism

_____ enuresis

a. pertaining to daytime or waking hours

b. attributing lifelike qualities to inanimate objects

c. concentrating on a single aspect of an object

d. involuntary urination after the age at which bladder control should have been established

e. viewing everything in reference to oneself

f. belief that everything is created by people

2. State the following typical vital signs in the preschool child.

   a. Pulse: ______ to ______ beats/minute

   b. Respirations: ______ breaths/minute

   c. Blood pressure: ______ systolic and ______ diastolic

3. Describe the following general characteristics of the three-year-old child.

   a. Sentences are ______________________________ than at age two and they can express ______________________ and ask ______________________________.

   b. They play __________________________ for short periods of time.

   c. May have a ________________________________ attachment to the parent of the opposite sex.

4. List three characteristics typical of the three-year-old child that contribute to fearfulness.

   a. ______________________________

   b. ______________________________

   c. ______________________________

5. Describe the following general characteristics of the four-year-old child.

   a. Prefers ______________________ toys.

   b. Plays with friends of the ______________ sex.

6. The four-year-old child is ______________ and likes to ______________.

7. Describe the following general characteristics of the five-year-old child.

   a. May begin losing ______________ teeth.

   b. Enjoys games that have ______________________.

8. Describe three ways children benefit from having limits set on their behavior.

   a. ______________________________

   ____

   ____

   b. ______________________________

   ____

   ____

   c. ______________________________

   ____

   ____

9. Good discipline is designed to shift responsibility for control from the ______________ to control by the ______________.

10. List three discipline methods that are often effective for the preschool child.

    a. ______________________________

    ____

    ____

Student Name ____________________

b. ____________________

____

____

c. ____________________

____

____

11. Masturbation in the preschool child is considered ____________________.

12. Describe the two types of enuresis (bedwetting).

    a. Primary ____________________

    b. Secondary ____________________

13. List seven possible causes of enuresis.

    a. ____________________

    b. ____________________

    c. ____________________

    d. ____________________

    e. ____________________

    f. ____________________

    g. ____________________

14. The ____________________ age of the child rather than the ____________________ age of the child should be considered when selecting toys for the child.

15. Hospitalization can be frightening to the preschool child because they are ____________________ and tend to be ____________________.

16. Preschool children cannot fully understand cause and effect and they may perceive illness and hospitalization as ____________________ for past behavior.

THINKING CRITICALLY

1. What are appropriate ways to encourage a preschool child's desire to do things for him- or herself while he or she is hospitalized in your clinical facility?

2. How would you help parents with the following common concerns about their preschool child?

    a. Use of bad language

    b. Thumb sucking

CASE STUDY

1. Sharon Giles is being discharged from the birth center with her second baby. Her three-year-old son Shawn has visited with her and the baby for several hours since the baby's birth. Sharon expresses concern about Shawn's relationship with the new baby since he has previously been the only child in the home. What guidance should the nurse give Sharon about minimizing Shawn's jealousy during the first few weeks after she and the baby go home?

OTHER LEARNING ACTIVITIES

1. As you care for children in the clinical area, identify examples of egocentrism, animism, and artificialism in their behavior.

2. Does your clinical facility have classes for siblings when a new baby is expected? What is included in the classes?

3. What kinds of nursery schools are available in your area? Are there publicly supported nursery schools for children who are from low-income families?

4. When you care for hospitalized children, are you able to use role modeling to teach parents? If you have not used role modeling, think of appropriate ways to use this parent teaching technique.

5. If your clinical facility has a play therapist, observe this staff member's work with children.

Student Name ____________________

REVIEW QUESTIONS

1. A preschool child falls off the swing and cries, "Bad swing! You made me fall!" This child's response is an example of
   a. egocentrism.
   b. intuition.
   c. animism.
   d. symbolism.

2. Choose the best example of egocentric thinking.
   a. "The airplane takes me to Grandma's."
   b. "Water is blue because someone colored it."
   c. "This big box is a truck."
   d. "The moon sleeps during the daytime."

3. Fears of preschool children are usually
   a. similar to those of older children.
   b. a result of the child's easy distraction.
   c. less intense than when they were younger.
   d. greater than those they had as toddlers.

4. Favorite stories of preschool children are those that relate to their
   a. aggressive tendencies.
   b. self-centeredness.
   c. daily experiences.
   d. relationships with others.

5. A healthy preschool girl asks her parents if she will die. The best response is to tell her that
   a. people do not usually die until they are old.
   b. she does not need to worry about dying.
   c. parents usually die before their children.
   d. she will not die for a long time.

6. The best way for parents to handle masturbation is to
   a. remove the child's hands from the genitals.
   b. try to interest the child in another activity.
   c. tell the child not to touch himself there.
   d. ask the child why he is rubbing that area.

7. One effective method of discipline for a preschool child is to
   a. reward the child for good behavior.
   b. give the child a light spanking.
   c. review the reasons for discipline.
   d. stop interacting with the child.

8. Choose the most effective way for parents to deal with a preschool child's jealousy of her new brother.
   a. Help her choose toys to share with the new baby.
   b. Remind her of things she can do that the baby cannot.
   c. Explain that she will soon love her new brother.
   d. Ask her to share her room with the new baby at first.

9. A child who sucks his thumb is unlikely to have damage to the mouth if the thumb sucking stops before
   a. three years of age.
   b. speech is established.
   c. the first teeth erupt.
   d. the permanent teeth erupt.

10. Choose the most appropriate teaching for parents of a child with enuresis.
    a. Girls tend to have the problem because they have smaller bladders.
    b. Most cases do not involve any abnormality and resolve without treatment.
    c. Limiting the child's fluid intake to body requirements usually resolves the problem.
    d. Most cases are the result of a minor urinary tract infection that is treatable.

11. Parents who send their child to a preschool program should expect their child to develop
    a. advanced academic skills for his/her age.
    b. control over expression of his/her feelings.
    c. self-confidence and a positive self-esteem.
    d. increased identification of unsafe behavior.

12. To foster normal personal and social development, it is best if children's regular playmates are
    a. about the same age they are.
    b. children with siblings.
    c. limited to one or two at a time.
    d. less aggressive than they are.

13. Play for mentally retarded children must specifically consider their
    a. tendency to become distracted.
    b. physical size and mental age.
    c. limited strength for their age.
    d. shyness around other children.

14. Delays or problems with language expression should be referred
    a. before five years of age.
    b. after completion of first grade.
    c. to a psychiatrist.
    d. only if the child has other delays.

15. Which type of play is imitative?
    a. "Reads" from a story book that he/she has heard many times.
    b. Says, "I'll be the mommy and you be the daddy."
    c. Climbs up and down a jungle gym.
    d. Participates in simple games with other children.

16. Choose the approximate age when children begin playing games that have simple rules.
    a. Three years
    b. Four years
    c. Five years
    d. Six years

17. Bedtime for the preschool child should include
    a. flexibility in the time the child goes to bed.
    b. a period of exercise after dinner.
    c. warm milk.
    d. a quiet activity such as a story.

Student Name ____________________

18. A major cause of health problems in preschool children is
    a. immunization reactions.
    b. communicable diseases.
    c. environmental allergies.
    d. accidental injuries.

chapter **19**

The School Age Child

LEARNING ACTIVITIES

1. Match the terms in the left column with their definitions on the right (a–d).

_____ concrete operations

_____ androgynous

_____ latchkey child

_____ preadolescent

a. period immediately preceding adolescence

b. sex role concept that incorporates both masculine and feminine qualities

c. logical thinking and an understanding of cause and effect

d. unsupervised children left at home after school

2. The school-age child differs from the preschool child in that he/she is more interested in ______________________________ than in fantasy.

3. Give approximate vital sign ranges for the school-age child.

   a. Pulse: ___________ to ___________ bpm

   b. Respiratory rate: ___________ to ___________ breaths/minute

   c. Systolic blood pressure: ___________ to ___________ mmHg

   d. Diastolic blood pressure: ___________ to ___________ mmHg

4. Describe information school-age children need in preparation for puberty.

   a. Boys ____

   ____

   b. Girls ____

   ____

Student Name ______________________________

5. Describe the following typical characteristics of a six-year-old child.

   a. The attention span is ______________________________.

   b. Loss of ______________________________ teeth occurs, along with eruption of ______________________________.

   c. Greater exposure to ______________________________ occurs with entry into school.

6. The seven-year-old child preferes toys that are ______________________________ ______________________________.

7. Describe the following typical characteristics of an eight-year-old child.

   a. Prefers friends of the ______________________________.

   b. Enjoys ______________________________ sports, but is a ______________________________.

   c. Secret clubs have strict ______________________________.

8. Describe the following typical characteristics of a nine-year-old child.

   a. ______________________________ and ______________________________ ______________________________ are common behaviors.

   b. ______________________________ sports are popular.

9. Describe the following typical characteristics of a 10-year-old preadolescent.

   a. Strives for ______________________________, but will take suggestions.

   b. Ideas of the ______________________________ are more important than those of the individual.

   c. Takes greater interest in his/her ______________________________.

10. Describe the following typical characteristics of 11- and 12-year-old preadolescents.

   a. This period is one of complete ______________________________.

   b. Has less ability to ______________________________.

   c. Has ______________________________ permanent teeth.

THINKING CRITICALLY

1. For each category listed below, describe one or two ways the nurse can incorporate the needs of the school-age child into care during hospitalization.
   a. Encouraging decision-making
   b. Need for inclusion in a group

CASE STUDIES

1. Rebecca, five years old, is receiving her booster immunizations before starting school. Her mother is concerned about how Rebecca will adjust to school because it is the first time she will be away from home for a significant part of the day. How can you help her mother prepare Rebecca for school?

2. Kyle, 10 years old, is hospitalized in skeletal traction with a badly fractured wrist and humerus that he suffered when playing street hockey with his friends. Kyle says he is really unhappy about being away from his friends during summer vacation. The boys spend most of the warm hours of the day at the public pool, and either skate or ride their bikes until dark. What safety teaching does Kyle need? How can you use knowledge of preadolescent growth and development to teach Kyle and his family about safety? What can you do to meet his needs for companionship with his friends?

OTHER LEARNING ACTIVITIES

1. Observe how experienced nurses prepare children of different ages for medical procedures. Identify ways they use knowledge of growth and development when caring for children of different ages but with similar medical conditions.

2. Watch television programs and evaluate them critically for positive and potentially harmful influences on children. Consider the following factors:
   a. Stimulating the child's imagination
   b. Materialistic focus
   c. Stereotypes (gender, age, race, and family structure)
   d. Violent content

Student Name ____________________

REVIEW QUESTIONS

1. The school-age child who has few experiences of success is likely to develop a sense of
   a. dependence.
   b. inferiority.
   c. trust.
   d. industry.

2. Which best describes physical growth of the school-age child?
   a. Rapid growth occurs from six to nine years of age, then slows.
   b. Slow growth continues until just before puberty.
   c. Height increases faster than weight.
   d. Height and weight remain stable until the onset of puberty.

3. Choose the normal characteristics of vital signs that the nurse should expect when assessing a nine-year-old girl.
   a. Blood pressure and pulse are higher than those of boys the same age.
   b. Blood pressure, pulse, and respirations are close to adult levels.
   c. Blood pressure is higher, but pulse and respirations are lower than the adult.
   d. Blood pressure, pulse, and respirations are higher than those of a six-year-old girl.

4. The best way to teach a child about sex is
   a. before they ask any questions.
   b. at their level of understanding.
   c. as part of the school curriculum.
   d. using terms used in the peer group.

5. The safest way for a child to cook is with a
   a. rice steamer.
   b. toaster oven.
   c. slow cooker.
   d. microwave oven.

6. The most significant physical development at six years is
   a. loss of the temporary teeth.
   b. elongation of the face.
   c. better infection resistance.
   d. rapid growth in height.

7. The school-age child who steals often does so because he
   a. does not understand that stealing is wrong.
   b. needs acceptance by his peer group.
   c. is rebelling against family expectations.
   d. is too young to earn his own spending money.

8. Worries and minor compulsions are more common at the age of
   a. 6 years.
   b. 7 years.
   c. 9 years.
   d. 11 years.

9. A preadolescent is more likely to accept her parents' decision if
   a. she understands why her parents made the decision.
   b. the parents do not change decisions once they are made.
   c. the parents carefully control the child's friends.
   d. her friends have values similar to her own family's.

10. Choose the most appropriate safety teaching related to a seven-year-old child's use of a bicycle.
    a. Use auxiliary ("training") wheels until balance is well-established.
    b. Select a well-fitting helmet in the child's choice of color and design.
    c. Restrict riding to light- or moderate-traffic streets near home.
    d. Do not allow the child to ride with friends who might distract him/her.

11. The preadolescent girl should have supplies for menstruation
    a. before her first menstrual period.
    b. as soon as she knows how heavy her flow is.
    c. when her friends are prepared for theirs.
    d. about six months after breast development begins.

12. Which characteristic is typical of many nine-year-old children?
    a. Enjoys secret codes and rituals with friends.
    b. Starts projects, but rarely completes them.
    c. Participates in intense teasing of the opposite sex.
    d. Argues and is bossy toward other children.

13. A group of eight- and nine-year-old boys has formed a "club." The boys have a secret password and handshake before they will meet. Parents should interpret this behavior as
    a. typical for children in this age group.
    b. a way to avoid being around adults.
    c. preceding criminal-type gang membership.
    d. rebellion against bossy older children.

14. A father is concerned because his nine-year-old son has developed the habit of wrinkling his nose unconsciously. The nurse should tell the father that his son
    a. may have a nerve problem and should be seen by a physician.
    b. cannot get adequate adult attention without taking this action.
    c. is probably doing this because of unresolved tension.
    d. should be corrected any time he is caught doing this action.

15. A school-age child has an adult "hero" of the same sex. What is the most appropriate interpretation of this behavior?
    a. The child feels insecure and inadequate around other children.
    b. Identifying with adults of the same sex is common at this time.
    c. Molestation or sexual abuse by the adult should be considered.
    d. The child is exploring various career and lifestyle options.

Student Name ____

chapter **20**

The Adolescent

LEARNING ACTIVITIES

1. Match the terms in the left column with their definitions on the right (a–h).

_____ adolescence
_____ androgens
_____ egocentrism
_____ estrogens
_____ menarche
_____ puberty
_____ growth spurt
_____ self-concept

a. one's view of oneself
b. rapid period of growth in which a body reaches adult height and weight
c. first menstrual period
d. period during which reproductive organs become functional
e. female sex hormones
f. male sex hormones
g. period beginning with appearance of secondary sex characteristics and ending with physical and emotional maturity
h. self-centeredness

2. Puberty occurs earliest in which gender? ____________________

3. Adolescents who engage in high-level physical activity may experience ________________________________.

4. The first change of puberty in a boy is ____________________________ ________________________________.

5. Boys begin sperm production at about ______________ years of age.

6. Two important cancer detection tests that are appropriately taught during adolescence are the ____________________________ and ____________________________ self-examinations.

7. Define *preadolescence.*

____

____

____

____

____

____

8. ____ is required for the adolescent to establish his/her own identity.

9. Describe several possible adult outcomes if the adolescent does not achieve his/her own identity.

____

____

____

____

10. Interpreting what is heard or seen literally is called ______________ thinking. The adolescent usually progresses toward the higher level of ______________ thinking.

11. State ways parents can help their teenager develop increased responsibility in each of these areas.

    a. Routine tasks ____

    ____

    ____

    b. Managing money ____

    ____

    ____

12. List two factors that increase the risk for nutritional deficiencies during adolescence.

    a. ____

    ____

    b. ____

    ____

Student Name ____

13. Why do adolescents need increased amounts of the following minerals?

    a. Calcium ____

    ____

    ____

    b. Iron (boys and girls) ____

    ____

    ____

14. The primary safety risk to the adolescent is related to use of a(n) ____.

15. Psychosocial milestones that must be accomplished during adolescence include the five "I"s.

    a. ____

    b. ____

    c. ____

    d. ____

    e. ____

16. A change in school performance, appearance, and behavior can be a warning sign of ______________________.

THINKING CRITICALLY

1. How might you best teach good nutrition compatible with her lifestyle to a teenage girl who is worried about being too "fat?"

2. A 16-year-old female confides in you that she is pregnant but does not want her parents to know. How would you respond?

CASE STUDIES

1. John's mother is worried about the change for the worse in the behavior of her only child. "Our family has always enjoyed many activities together, but now John only wants to be with his friends. He doesn't seem to care that his clothes look bizarre, and yet he's constantly fussing with his hair. He never seems to pay attention. I'm afraid his grades will fall and he won't get into a good college." Can you help John's mother understand his behavior? What guidance might be appropriate for her?

2. Mary Lou, 15 years old, confides to you that she and her boyfriend have had sex a few times. Mary Lou is concerned about getting pregnant, but does not know much about contraception. She says that talking to her parents about sex and contraception is out of the question. How can you help Mary Lou make responsible decisions concerning her sexuality? What problems have you seen in adolescents who become parents?

OTHER LEARNING ACTIVITIES

1. Observe a group of young adolescents. Identify behaviors in the group that demonstrate the following.
   a. Efforts to develop an identity
   b. Preoccupation with self
   c. Cultural variations

2. Obtain statistics for your state and city about the number of vehicle accidents in which teenagers were involved. If possible, determine how long the young drivers had been licensed.

3. Visit community groups that focus on reducing gang violence among teenagers. Determine the approximate ages of gang members and how they identify themselves to one another and to rival gangs.

4. Obtain local statistics for violent deaths among teenagers. How many of these are thought to be related to gangs?

REVIEW QUESTIONS

1. Younger adolescents often have an awkward appearance because
   a. maturation occurs earlier than in previous generations.
   b. body parts grow and mature at different rates.
   c. growth and development slows during adolescence.
   d. self-consciousness causes the adolescent to slump.

2. A person who does not establish an identity during adolescence is more likely to
   a. conform to a peer group for a prolonged time.
   b. seek close relationships with others.
   c. become insensitive to the needs of others.
   d. have an overly superior self-image.

3. A parent can best help an adolescent make a wise decision by
   a. explaining what he/she would have done when he/she was a teenager.
   b. reviewing problems with the decision after the teenager makes it.
   c. serving as a role model by making the decision for the teenager.
   d. respecting the teenager's decision, even if he/she makes a mistake.

Student Name ____________________

4. Younger adolescents tend to be egocentric because they are

   a. certain that their parents are ignorant.

   b. believe no-one is paying attention to them.

   c. preoccupied with their physical development.

   d. proud of their greater responsibilities.

5. The adolescent's peer group helps him/her move away from

   a. same-sex friendships.

   b. values of his/her family.

   c. individual responsibility.

   d. dependence on his/her family.

6. Daydreaming in the adolescent should be interpreted as a

   a. normal occurrence.

   b. sign of insecurity.

   c. symptom of depression.

   d. desire to ignore parents.

7. Adolescents have high calcium needs because of their rapidly increasing

   a. blood volume.

   b. muscle mass.

   c. bone growth.

   d. sexual maturity.

8. An adolescent who adopts a strict vegetarian diet is at risk for a deficiency of

   a. calcium.

   b. vitamin C.

   c. protein.

   d. fiber.

9. Most accidents in adolescence occur when they

   a. participate in contact sports.

   b. handle guns or knives.

   c. drive a car or other vehicle.

   d. work at part-time jobs.

10. Greater intake of iron is important to adolescents of both sexes primarily because of

    a. a more rapid rate of red blood cell breakdown.

    b. growth in muscle and bone and because of menstrual losses.

    c. inadequate intake of foods high in vitamin C.

    d. reduced storage of the mineral in the liver.

11. Tanner stages describe the

    a. sequence of physical maturation in the adolescent.

    b. change from concrete thinking to abstract thinking.

    c. hormonal changes that cause ovulation and menstruation.

    d. development of a mature gender identity.

12. The major psychosocial task of adolescence is to develop a sense of

    a. sexual orientation.

    b. concern for other people.

    c. family unity.

    d. identity as an individual.

13. The most important teaching for an adolescent with body piercing is to

    a. apply an antibiotic cream daily.

    b. change the body ring daily.

    c. not share body rings with others.

    d. avoid placing the hands near the pierced area.

14. A woman is worried because her 14-year-old son seems to be constantly in the bathroom, shampooing and styling his hair. She worries that her son may be homosexual because he is so concerned about his appearance. Choose the best counseling for this mother.

    a. Homosexual thoughts and experimentation are normal during the early teens.

    b. Boys are usually more concerned about their athletic abilities than their appearance.

    c. She should be more concerned about why he does not want to be with his friends.

    d. Teens are preoccupied with their appearance because of dramatic body changes.

15. The most important consideration when teaching a teenager about a healthy diet is to

    a. include information about nourishing foods at fast-food restaurants.

    b. focus primarily on nutrients that are most often deficient in a teenage diet.

    c. teach the importance of an adequate diet to better health during adulthood.

    d. explain that dieting during adolescence can result in lifetime weight-control problems.

Student Name ______________________________

chapter **21**

The Child's Experience of Hospitalization

LEARNING ACTIVITIES

1. Match the terms in the left column with their definitions on the right (a–d).

_____ clinical pathway	a. brothers and sisters
_____ emancipated minor	b. loss of an achieved level of functioning to a past level of behavior
_____ regression	c. interdisciplinary plan of care that displays progress of the treatment plan for a patient
_____ siblings	d. adolescent younger than 18 years of age who is no longer under the parents' authority

2. How can the trauma associated with giving a five-month-old infant an injection be decreased?

____

____

3. List three examples of transitional objects that can be brought to the hospital for a nine-month-old child.

a. ______________________________

b. ______________________________

c. ______________________________

4. List three ways the nurse can decrease the anxiety of siblings when a brother or sister is hospitalized.

a. ______________________________

____

b. ______________________________

____

c. ______________________________

____

5. Give two methods of decreasing the stress of hospitalization for an infant.

a. ______________________________

b. ______________________________

6. Identify and describe the three stages of separation anxiety.

a. ______________________________

____

b. ______________________________

____

c. ______________________________

____

7. List three nonpharmacologic methods of pain reduction.

a. ______________________________

b. ______________________________

c. ______________________________

8. Explain how the nurse would prepare a preschool child for abdominal surgery.

____

____

____

9. Give three examples of nonverbal clues that school-age children experiencing pain might exhibit.

a. ______________________________

b. ______________________________

c. ______________________________

Student Name ______________________________

10. List four nursing interventions for the child in pain.

    a. ______________________________

    b. ______________________________

    c. ______________________________

    d. ______________________________

11. Illness in the young adolescent is seen mainly as a threat to ______________________________.

12. Following treatments, what should the nurse encourage the school-age child to do? ______________________________

13. List four advantages of outpatient surgery for the pediatric patient.

    a. ______________________________

    b. ______________________________

    c. ______________________________

    d. ______________________________

14. The child's reaction to hospitalization depends on:

    a. ______________________________
    ____

    b. ______________________________
    ____

    c. ______________________________
    ____

    d. ______________________________
    ____

    e. ______________________________
    ____

15. List three things the nurse can do to lesson anxiety in the parents of a hospitalized child.

    a. ______________________________

    ____

    b. ______________________________

    ____

    c. ______________________________

    ____

16. What is the major issue affecting the adolescent who is hospitalized?

    ____

17. What should be included in the documentation when a child is discharged?

    a. ______________________________

    b. ______________________________

    c. ______________________________

    d. ______________________________

    e. ______________________________

18. List four suggestions the nurse can give parents who are concerned about behavioral problems arising with their children after hospitalization.

    a. ______________________________

    ____

    b. ______________________________

    ____

    c. ______________________________

    ____

    d. ______________________________

    ____

THINKING CRITICALLY

1. Prepare a care plan for a hospitalized toddler. Address the psychosocial needs of the child and parents. Include nursing diagnoses, goals, and interventions.

Student Name ____________________

2. Do you think parents have the right to know if their children are being treated for a sexually transmitted disease? Discuss this with your classmates.

CASE STUDY

1. Scott, age six months, is admitted to the hospital with a diagnosis of croup. He has an IV infusing and is in a mist tent. Both of his parents work, as well as care for two older siblings.
   a. Scott's mother confides to the nurse that she feels that this hospitalization could have been avoided if she would have taken Scott to the doctor sooner. How can the nurse best answer the mother?
   b. Scott's parents take turns spending the night with Scott but are unable to be with him during the day. What fears and behaviors might the parents show because of their separation from Scott?
   c. When assessing Scott's IV, the nurse should make what observations in her charting?
   d. What are four nursing interventions the nurse would use with Scott because he is in an oxygen tent?

OTHER LEARNING ACTIVITIES

1. Involve a school-age child in a board game. What type of communication were you able to develop using this strategy?
2. While you are in the clinical area, assess a toddler who is alone for signs of separation anxiety. What stage is this child in?
3. Take a hospitalized child to the playroom. Compare the child's behavior while in the playroom to behavior in the hospital room.
4. Discuss with your peers how you feel when parents do not come to visit their hospitalized child. What could be some reasons for their not visiting?
5. Determine the laws in your state governing the treatment of minors.

REVIEW QUESTIONS

1. Separation anxiety is most pronounced in which age group?
   a. infants
   b. toddlers
   c. preschool children
   d. adolescents

2. The mother of a hospitalized toddler could best explain when she will return by saying
   a. "I will be back in three hours."
   b. "I will be back after your nap."
   c. "I will be back before six o'clock."
   d. "I will be back before you know it."

3. In most instances, unpleasant treatments on children should take place in the
   a. playroom.
   b. emergency room.
   c. patient's room.
   d. treatment room.

4. A child who is anxious about hospitalization will probably benefit most from
   a. a visit from Bozo the clown.
   b. having her favorite toy brought from home.
   c. having her favorite foods served at lunch.
   d. opening a new gift each day.

5. Children in which of these age groups would most likely feel their illness is punishment for something they have done wrong?
   a. toddler
   b. preschool child
   c. school-age child
   d. adolescent

6. Anxiety over surgery can sometimes be decreased by
   a. not telling the child that he/she is having surgery.
   b. allowing the child to meet the surgeon.
   c. visiting the surgical area preoperatively.
   d. riding on the stretcher before surgery.

7. Parental consent for minors is not always necessary for the treatment of
   a. minor cuts and abrasions.
   b. psychologic disorders.
   c. communicable diseases.
   d. sexually transmitted diseases.

8. The nurse notices that the mother of a child with cerebral palsy always corrects and redoes many of things the nurse does for her child. The best response to the mother would be
   a. "Would you like to do all of Jimmy's care?"
   b. "I'm doing the best I can."
   c. "You are going to be exhausted if you don't go home."
   d. "I'd be happy if you would share with me some of the special things you do with Jimmy."

9. The mother of three-year-old Jason is concerned because he has returned to diapers since he has been hospitalized although he had been potty trained. What should the nurse say to the mother?
   a. "This is very unusual and I'm sure it is temporary."
   b. "Keep him in his training pants and don't give in to him."
   c. "Regression is normal in a sick child."
   d. "Perhaps he has some type of urinary infection."

10. The nurse's best approach to prepare a toddler for a painful procedure is to
   a. be truthful if it will be painful.
   b. avoid frightening him by telling him it might hurt.
   c. begin preparing early so that he can ask questions.
   d. have his mother explain what will happen.

Student Name ______________________________

11. The mother of a small child disciplines him when he protests before a procedure. The nurse's best approach with this mother is to
    a. realize that disciplining the child is her right.
    b. explain that this is the child's way of relieving tension.
    c. ask the mother to leave the room.
    d. assist the mother in trying to keep the child quiet.

12. Hospitalized school-age children who act out should be
    a. placed in a private room.
    b. disciplined by having restrictions put in place.
    c. provided with positive direction and consistency.
    d. ignored because this is a normal reaction to hospitalization.

13. After performing a painful procedure on an infant, the nurse should
    a. swaddle the infant.
    b. feed the infant.
    c. return the infant to the parent.
    d. change the infant's diaper.

14. A toddler ignores his mother when she comes for a visit. The child
    a. has adjusted to hospitalization.
    b. is coping by detaching.
    c. has a poor mother-child relationship.
    d. is bored.

15. A common reaction of the preschooler to hospitalization is
    a. anger.
    b. depression.
    c. guilt.
    d. fear.

16. The hospitalized adolescent should be allowed to participate in his/her own care in order to
    a. decrease fear of bodily injury.
    b. increase self-esteem.
    c. allow some control.
    d. increase responsibility.

17. The mother of a hospitalized child states, "He cries when I visit. I should just stay away!" What would be the nurse's best response?
    a. "Perhaps you are right, since he becomes so upset when you come."
    b. "I can't make that decision for you."
    c. "It's up to you, but we can take good care of him and he seems fine when you are not here."
    d. "It is important that you be here. This is a common reaction in children when they are separated from their parents."

18. An adolescent who refuses to keep a record of his intake and output may be dealing with issues of
    a. separation.
    b. control.
    c. self-esteem.
    d. body image.

19. Because of distance, the family of a six-year-old child cannot be at the hospital with her. The nurse suggests that the family
    a. hire a private duty nurse.
    b. bring in photographs and special toys.
    c. not tell the child that they will not be visiting.
    d. not call the child because it would be upsetting.

20. Taking blood pressure can be upsetting to a toddler. The nurse can decrease anxiety by

    a. taking the blood pressure while the child is sleeping.

    b. asking the mother to take the blood pressure.

    c. demonstrating the procedure on the child's doll prior to doing it to the child.

    d. telling the child that big boys/girls do not cry when they have their blood pressure taken.

Student Name ______________________________

chapter **22**

Health Care Adaptations for the Child and Family

LEARNING ACTIVITIES

1. Match the acronyms in the left column with their definitions on the right (a–d).

_____ O.D.	a. right eye
_____ O.S.	b. both eyes
_____ O.U.	c. total parenteral nutrition or hyperalimentation
_____ T.P.N.	d. left eye

2. List six safety measures applicable to the hospitalized child.

a. ______________________________

b. ______________________________

c. ______________________________

d. ______________________________

e. ______________________________

f. ______________________________

3. What are four safety hazards to avoid when caring for a hospitalized child?

   a. ______________________________

   ____

   b. ______________________________

   ____

   c. ______________________________

   ____

   d. ______________________________

   ____

4. One of the most important initial observations a nurse can make when assessing a child's mental status is to determine if the child is ________ and ______________ to the environment.

5. A ______________ fontanelle may indicate dehydration and a ____________ fontanelle may indicate increased intracranial pressure.

6. *Fever* is defined as a temperature over ________ F/________ C in infants under three months or above ________ F/________ C in children over three months.

7. Apical pulses are advised for children under age _______ years and should be counted for ____________ seconds.

8. The width of the blood pressure cuff should cover _________________ of the upper arm.

9. A rectal thermometer should be inserted a maximum of ________ inch(es).

10. The preferred method of obtaining a child's temperature is ___________ or ____________________.

11. Describe the ultrasonographic measurement of blood pressure.

____

____

____

____

____

Student Name ______________________________

12. Describe the procedure for weighing an infant.

____
____
____
____
____
____

13. Describe the procedure for collecting a urine specimen from an infant.

____
____
____
____
____

14. What is the purpose of a lumbar puncture?

____
____

15. Explain how a nurse should position a child for a lumbar puncture.

____
____
____
____
____

16. What information should be recorded after a lumbar puncture?

____
____
____

17. What is the most common way to calculate a safe dosage when administering medications to children?

____

____

18. Give the calculation that uses body surface area (BSA) to determine a safe medication dosage.

____

____

____

____

19. Describe the procedure for administering medication to an infant with an oral syringe.

____

____

____

20. Compare the procedure for administering ear drops to children under three years of age and children three years of age and older.

____

____

____

____

____

21. ____________________, ____________________, and ____________________ catheters are tiny, flexible rubber tubes inserted into a vein in the chest to establish long-term intravenous therapy.

22. When intravenous fluids are infusing, the nurse observes the child for

a. ____

b. ____

c. ____

d. ____

e. ____

Student Name ____________________

23. Total parenteral nutrition is given to children who ____________________
____________________.

24. Describe the procedure for giving a gastrostomy tube feeding.

____

____

____

____

____

25. When administering an enema to a child, the __________, __________, and the __________ of insertion of the tube require modification.

26. Why is it necessary to add moisture and humidity to the room of a child with a tracheostomy?

____

____

27. List four indications that suctioning is needed.

a. ____________________

b. ____________________

c. ____________________

d. ____________________

28. Describe the procedure for suctioning a child with a tracheostomy.

____

____

____

____

____

____

29. Describe the care of the tracheal stoma and the changing of the tape around the child's neck.

____

____

____

____

____

____

____

30. List six of the signs and symptoms that might indicate a problem in a tracheostomy patient.

    a. ____

    b. ____

    c. ____

    d. ____

    e. ____

    f. ____

31. What emergency equipment should be kept at the bedside of a tracheotomy patient?

____

32. What should be included in the documentation when assessing a child with a tracheotomy?

    a. ____

    b. ____

    c. ____

    d. ____

    e. ____

33. Prior to surgery, infants should not be maintained on NPO status longer than _____ to _________ hours because of the risk of _______________________.

Student Name ____

THINKING CRITICALLY

1. You are assisting a registered nurse who is going to start intravenous fluids on a three-month-old infant. The mother is crying and is not sure if she wants to be with the infant or to remain outside the room during the procedure. How could you support this mother?

OTHER LEARNING ACTIVITIES

1. Where would the following items and areas be found in the clinical setting?
   a. Blood pressure machine
   b. Diapers
   c. Emergency cart
   d. Intake and output sheet
   e. IV soluset
   f. Oral medication syringe
   g. Playroom
   h. Procedure manual
   i. Scales
   j. Thermometer
   l. Treatment room
   k. Urine collection bag
2. Assist a registered nurse when she starts an IV on a child.
3. Care for a child with a tracheotomy tube.
4. Care for a child in an oxygen tent.
5. Care for a child with an IV infusing.

REVIEW QUESTIONS

1. Pulse and respiration rates of children are
   a. lower than adults.
   b. the same as adults.
   c. higher than adults.
   d. lower at birth, but higher by age three years.

2. Unpleasant-tasting medications can be mixed in
   a. orange juice.
   b. milk.
   c. jelly.
   d. cereal.

3. An infant's diaper weighs 30 g. How many milliliters would you record on the intake and output sheet?

   a. 15

   b. 30

   c. 60

   d. 45

4. When caring for a tracheotomy patient, the nurse should

   a. limit suctioning to 30–40 seconds.

   b. insert the catheter the length of the tracheotomy tube and no more than 0.5 cm beyond the tube.

   c. replace suctioning catheters every 12 hours and if they are dropped.

   d. replace water used to clear catheter at the end of the shift.

5. In giving a child a sponge bath to reduce body temperature, the nurse should

   a. continue sponging the child until the temperature is within normal limits.

   b. use a mixture of half water and half alcohol.

   c. keep the body uncovered to increase evaporation.

   d. use tepid water.

6. An infant should be weighed

   a. completely naked.

   b. with a diaper in place.

   c. wrapped in a receiving blanket.

   d. completely dressed.

7. The neonate exposed to prolonged high oxygen concentrations is at risk for damage to the

   a. heart.

   b. lungs.

   c. brain.

   d. kidneys.

8. Both the pulse and respirations of children should be counted for _____ seconds.

   a. 15

   b. 30

   c. 45

   d. 60

9. The blood pressure cuff on a child's upper arm should cover

   a. one-half of the upper arm.

   b. one-third of the upper arm.

   c. two-thirds of the upper arm.

   d. the entire upper arm.

10. The acronym O.D. refers to the

    a. right eye.

    b. right ear.

    c. left eye.

    d. left ear.

11. The preferred injection site for infants is the

    a. deltoid.

    b. ventrogluteal.

    c. vastus lateralis.

    d. dorsogluteal.

12. The maximum volume that can be given by intramuscular injection at one site to older infants and small children is

    a. 0.1 ml.

    b. 0.5 ml.

    c. 1 ml.

    d. 1.1 ml.

Student Name ______________________________

13. Documentation on the child receiving IV fluids should occur
    a. every 15 minutes.
    b. every 30 minutes.
    c. hourly.
    d. every 4 hours.

14. After receiving a gastrostomy tube feeding, an infant should be placed in what position when returned to bed?
    a. left side
    b. supine
    c. right side
    d. prone

15. Which type of enema solution is contraindicated in infants and children?
    a. saline
    b. oil-retention
    c. tap water

16. When giving an enema to an infant, the tube should be inserted in
    a. 1/2 inch.
    b. 1 inch.
    c. 2 inches.
    d. 3 inches.

17. Children receiving opioid analgesic drugs should be observed closely for
    a. gastrointestinal upset.
    b. urinary retention.
    c. respiratory distress.
    d. blurred vision.

18. The ideal site for intravenous placement in the infant is the
    a. scalp.
    b. forearm.
    c. foot.
    d. hand.

chapter **23**

The Child with a Sensory or Neurological Condition

LEARNING ACTIVITIES

1. Match the terms in the left column with their definitions on the right (a–n).

_____ athetosis
_____ hyperopia
_____ hyphema
_____ myringotomy
_____ nystagmus
_____ opisthotonos
_____ otoscope
_____ papilledema
_____ postictal
_____ strabismus
_____ dyslexia
_____ concussion
_____ decerebrate
_____ decorticate

a. presence of blood in the anterior chamber of the eye
b. involuntary, purposeless movements
c. involuntary arching of the back and extension of the neck due to muscle contractions
d. reading disability that involves a defect in the cortex of the brain that processes graphic symbols
e. period following a seizure
f. farsighted
g. incision of the tympanic membrane
h. involuntary movement of the eye
i. instrument used to view the ear
j. edema and inflammation of the optic nerve
k. cross-eyed
l. temporary disturbance of the brain followed by a period of unconsciousness
m. rigid extension and pronation of the arms and legs
n. adduction of arms, flexed on chest with wrists flexed, hands fisted, lower extremities extended and adducted

Student Name ______________________________

2. Explain why infants are more prone to ear infections than older children.

____

____

____

3. List the main symptoms of otitis media.

____

____

4. List the three of the possible complications of otitis media.

   a. ______________________________

   b. ______________________________

   c. ______________________________

5. Describe the treatment of otitis media.

____

____

6. What teaching should be done when antibiotics are prescribed for children?

____

____

____

7. Describe some of the behavior problems that deaf children may experience.

____

____

____

____

____

8. Complete bilateral deafness is usually discovered during ________, but partial deafness may be unrecognized until ______________________.

9. List some common signs seen in infants and school-age children that might indicate a hearing problem.

Infants

a. ______________________________

b. ______________________________

School-age children

a. ______________________________

b. ______________________________

10. When caring for a hospitalized school-age child who is deaf, the nurse should

a. ______________________________

b. ______________________________

c. ______________________________

d. ______________________________

e. ______________________________

f. ______________________________

11. During a visual assessment, the nurse should observe the eyes for

a. ______________________________

b. ______________________________

12. Visual acuity can be tested by _______ to __________ years of age.

13. Symptoms of strabismus include

a. ______________________________

b. ______________________________

c. ______________________________

d. ______________________________

e. ______________________________

f. ______________________________

14. Untreated strabismus can result in ______________________________.

Student Name ______________________________

15. Explain the goal and treatment of amblyopia.

____
____
____
____
____

16. Why might a child be embarrassed when being treated for amblyopia?

____
____
____

17. Describe the procedure for wiping secretions from the eye in the child with conjunctivitis.

____
____

18. Neural tube development occurs about the ______________ to ______________ week of fetal life.

19. What medication, when used during a viral illness, has been linked to Reye's syndrome? ______________________________

20. Describe the signs and symptoms of a child with Reye's syndrome.

____
____
____
____

21. The peak incidence of bacterial meningitis is between what ages? ______________
____

22. List five signs and symptoms of meningitis.

a. ______________________________
b. ______________________________
c. ______________________________
d. ______________________________
e. ______________________________

23. Nursing measures for the child with meningitis include

    a. ______________________________

    b. ______________________________

    c. ______________________________

    d. ______________________________

24. List two measures the nurse should take to decrease stimuli when caring for a child with meningitis.

    a. ______________________________

    b. ______________________________

25. Preoperative care of a child with a brain tumor should address what body image issue? ______________________________

26. What is a series of convulsions rapidly following one another called?

    ____

27. What information should the nurse observe and record after a seizure?

    a. ______________________________

    b. ______________________________

    c. ______________________________

    d. ______________________________

    e. ______________________________

    f. ______________________________

    g. ______________________________

28. List four common causes of cerebral palsy.

    a. ______________________________

    b. ______________________________

    c. ______________________________

    d. ______________________________

Student Name ____________________

29. List three clinical manifestations that might indicate a child has cerebral palsy.

    a. ____________________

    b. ____________________

    c. ____________________

30. Interventions that can decrease the occurrence of mental retardation include

    a. ____________________

    b. ____________________

    c. ____________________

    d. ____________________

31. What are three problems associated with feeding a child with cerebral palsy?

    a. ____________________

    b. ____________________

    c. ____________________

32. List two approaches that parents of children who are mentally retarded can take to enhance their child's abilities.

    a. ____________________

    b. ____________________

33. Four components of a neurologic check are

    a. ____________________

    b. ____________________

    c. ____________________

    d. ____________________

34. List four major complications of head injuries.

    a. ____________________

    b. ____________________

    c. ____________________

    d. ____________________

35. List three questions you could ask a four-year-old child to help determine his/her level of consciousness.

    a. ______________________________

    b. ______________________________

    c. ______________________________

36. Name three things you could observe to test the motor ability of a child with a head injury.

    a. ______________________________

    b. ______________________________

    c. ______________________________

37. What special observations should be made of an infant with a head injury?

    a. ______________________________

    b. ______________________________

    c. ______________________________

THINKING CRITICALLY

1. Visit your local Easter Seal Society and observe the therapy of children with cerebral palsy. Find out what resources are available for these children.

CASE STUDIES

1. Six-year-old Christina is admitted to the hospital with Reye's syndrome. She is unconscious and is in the ICU.

    a. What nursing measures can the nurse perform that would be helpful to Christina's parents?

    b. What are two nursing diagnoses that would be appropriate for Christina?

    c. What are some specific nursing interventions for a child who is comatose?

2. Kevin, age six months, is admitted to the hospital with meningitis. He is placed in isolation, an IV is started, and he is on seizure precautions.

    a. What changes in Kevin's spinal fluid would confirm a diagnosis of meningitis?

    b. Kevin's temperature is 102.4° F. What other signs and symptoms would the nurse assess for?

    c. Give at least six nursing interventions for Kevin.

Student Name ______________________________

OTHER LEARNING ACTIVITIES

1. While in the clinical area, care for a child who is on seizure precautions. What are some of the special procedures you followed?

2. Observe the following in children in the clinical area.
   a. Reflexes of a newborn
   b. Gait
   c. Finger–nose test

3. Care for a child with meningitis. Observe for neurologic involvement.

4. Assist with vision screening in your local school district.

REVIEW QUESTIONS

1. Children with tympanostomy tubes should
   a. be given antibiotics.
   b. avoid getting water in their ears.
   c. sleep on their backs.
   d. take a decongestant.

2. Visual acuity can be checked by age
   a. 2 ½–3 years.
   b. 3–4 years.
   c. 4–5 years.
   d. 5–6 years.

3. Early signs of Reye's syndrome include
   a. diarrhea and headache.
   b. vomiting and lethargy.
   c. nausea and malaise.
   d. hyperactivity and vomiting.

4. When taking the history of a child with encephalitis, it is important to note recent
   a. cat scratches.
   b. tick bites.
   c. respiratory infection.
   d. drug therapy.

5. Cerebral palsy is
   a. a form of mental retardation that does not improve with treatment.
   b. a nonprogressive disorder that affects the motor centers of the brain.
   c. always caused by a birth injury occurring in early gestational births.
   d. related to lack of early childhood stimulation and is irreversible.

6. Children with cerebral palsy tend to
   a. tire easily.
   b. have short-term memory loss.
   c. have an increased appetite.
   d. thrive on overstimulation.

7. The most common causative agent of bacterial meningitis is
   a. *Haemophilus influenzae.*
   b. *Streptococcus pneumoniae.*
   c. *Neisseria meningitides.*
   d. *Escherichia coli.*

8. Which of the following are signs and symptoms of meningitis?
   a. diarrhea and stiff neck
   b. hyperactivity and vomiting
   c. irritability and fever
   d. loss of vision and nausea

9. A child with meningitis should be
   a. placed with another child his/her age.
   b. have vital signs checked every 15 minutes.
   c. be disturbed as little as possible.
   d. have levels of consciousness checked every 15 minutes.

10. Febrile seizures
    a. are common in newborns.
    b. are treated with alcohol baths.
    c. are usually controlled with Phenobarbital.
    d. rarely develop into epilepsy.

11. Fluids are monitored in children with a head injury in order to
    a. prevent renal damage.
    b. control cerebral edema.
    c. prevent aspiration.
    d. decrease headaches

12. Nursing care for a child experiencing a seizure should include
    a. attempting to hold the tongue.
    b. administration of oxygen.
    c. restraint.
    d. turning on his/her side.

13. A common side effect of Dilantin is
    a. drowsiness.
    b. gum overgrowth.
    c. hyperactivity.
    d. headache.

14. When caring for a hospitalized child who is deaf, the nurse should
    a. speak in a loud, clear tone.
    b. speak in separate words.
    c. speak in a clear, natural tone.
    d. speak in an exaggerated tone.

15. An infant brought to the emergency room with a high fever, irritability, and a high-pitched cry would immediately be evaluated for
    a. retinoblastoma.
    b. Reye's syndrome.
    c. neuroblastoma.
    d. meningitis.

16. An infant with bacterial meningitis should be
    a. restrained when awake.
    b. positioned on the right side.
    c. kept in a quiet, indirectly lit area.
    d. placed in isolation until discharged.

17. A child has a Glasgow Coma Scale score of 15. The nurse should
    a. tell the charge nurse immediately.
    b. change the position of the child.
    c. chart the results of the assessment.
    d. stimulate the child.

18. When caring for a child with a head injury, the nurse should
    a. force fluids.
    b. wake the child every hour.
    c. notify the physician if the child's blood pressure decreases.
    d. report any abnormal posturing.

Student Name ______________________________

19. Parents of a child with a head injury should be advised to call their primary caregiver if the child
    a. falls asleep.
    b. develops a bump.
    c. vomits one time.
    d. cannot be aroused.

20. Signs of impending increased intracranial pressure include
    a. dilated, sluggish pupils.
    b. constricted, sluggish pupils.
    c. constricted, hyperreactive pupils.
    d. dilated, hyperreactive pupils.

chapter **24**

The Child with a Musculoskeletal Condition

LEARNING ACTIVITIES

1. Match the terms in the left column with their definitions on the right (a–h).

A	arthroscope	a.	endoscope for examining interior of a joint
B	genu varum	b.	bow-legged or knees turned outward
E	iridocyclitis	c.	knock-kneed or knees turned inward
F	osteochondroses	d.	tearing of the collagenous fibers that connect muscle to bone
G	subluxation	e.	inflammation of the iris and ciliary body of eye
C	genu valgum	f.	disease affecting bone cartilage
D	shin splint	g.	incomplete dislocation

2. Assessment of the musculoskeletal system in children who can walk includes

a. Observation,

b. Palpation

c. ROM (range of motion)

d. Gait

3. List three types of traction used for children.

a. Bryant traction

b. Buck extension

c. Russell traction

Student Name Shirley Williams

4. The most common type of muscular dystrophy is Duchenne's muscular dystrophy.

5. List three signs that might indicate a child has muscular dystrophy.

   a. Progressive weakness, frequent falling

   b. The calf muscle become hypertrophied

   c. Clumsiness, contractures of the ankles & hips & the Gowers maneuver.

6. Describe the treatment of a soft tissue injury.

   A cold pack & elastic wrap will reduce edema, bleeding, relieve pain & should be applied @ alternating 30 min. intervals. After a 30 min. period ischemia can occur & that will impede the tissue perfusion

7. List two clinical manifestations of Legg-Calvé-Perthes disease.

   a. The marked distortion of the head of the femur may lead to an imperfect joint or

   b. degenerative arthritis.

8. What would you tell the parents about the prognosis of Legg-Calvé-Perthes disease in their child?

   I would them that its a self limiting disorder that heals spontaneously; & the treatment involves keeping the femoral head deep into the hip socket & no wt. bearing while healing.

9. Complete the following traction related statements.

   a. Weights are hanging freely.

   b. Weights are out of reach of child.

   c. Ropes are on the pulleys.

   d. Knots are not resting against pulleys.

   e. Bed linens are not on traction ropes.

   f. Countertraction is in place.

   g. Apparatus does not touch the foot of the bed.

10. Match the types of fractures in the left column with their definitions on the right (a–d).

B simple
C compound
A complete
D greenstick

a. bone is entirely broken across
b. bone is broken, but skin over area is not broken
c. open fracture in which the wound in the skin leads to the broken bone
d. incomplete fracture

11. Bryant traction is used for treating fractures of the femur in children under 2 years of age or under 20 to 30 pounds.

12. Explain Russell traction.
It's similar to the Buck Extension, in the former a sling is positioned under the knee, it suspends the distal thigh above the bed. Skin traction is applied to the lower extremity. It pulls in two directions, vertically from the knee sling + longitudinally from the footplate.

13. Children with skin traction have the added risk of developing a(n) __________.

14. Based on the signs and symptoms and treatment of osteomyelitis, list three appropriate nursing diagnoses for this disease.

a. __________

b. __________

c. __________

15. What are the goals of care of juvenile rheumatoid arthritis?

a. __________
b. __________
c. __________
d. __________
e. __________

Student Name ____

16. A neurovascular assessment of the toes of a child with a fracture who has a cast or ace bandage includes checking for

    a. ____

    b. ____

    c. ____

    d. ____

    e. ____

    f. ____

17. Define *compartment syndrome.*

    ____

    ____

18. The two types of scoliosis are ____________________ and ____________________.

19. The Milwaukee brace must be worn __________ hours a day.

20. Screening for scoliosis should be done before ____________________.

    What does a screening examination involve?

    ____

    ____

    ____

    ____

    ____

    ____

21. A child with scoliosis who needs a spinal fusion has special needs related to immobilization. What is the appropriate nursing diagnosis?

____

____

List the nursing care associated with immobility.

a. _______________

b. _______________

c. _______________

d. _______________

22. A parent asks you for guidelines to help prevent sports injuries in a child who is in competitive sports. List four guidelines.

a. _______________

b. _______________

c. _______________

d. _______________

23. Amenorrhea can be induced by _______________ _______________.

24. What is the treatment for shin splints?

____

____

25. When a nurse suspects child abuse he/she must _______________ _______________.

THINKING CRITICALLY

1. Identify three nursing diagnoses for an adolescent with juvenile rheumatoid arthritis who is being discharged from the hospital. Include psychological needs as well as physiologic.

2. Nurses who care for abused children may have negative feelings toward the adult who abused the child. Examine your thoughts on this issue. Discuss ways that you might provide nursing care for the child as well as the adult who abused the child. How will supporting the adult ultimately help the child?

Student Name ______________________________

CASE STUDY

1. Two-year-old Kimberly is admitted to the hospital with a fractured femur. She is placed in Bryant traction.
   a. Kimberly's mother asks why this particular type of traction is used. How should the nurse reply?
   b. What particular areas of Kimberly's body would be assessed? Provide rationales.
   c. What are some diversional activities the nurse could plan for the child? Base the plan on growth and development knowledge.

OTHER LEARNING ACTIVITIES

1. While in the clinical area, care for a child in traction or in a body cast.
2. Screen a 10-year-old girl for scoliosis.
3. While in the clinical area, care for a child with a head injury.
4. Label the following bones on Figure 24-1 of the textbook.
   a. Femur
   b. Tibia
   c. Fibula
   d. Ulna
   e. Radius
   f. Coccyx
   g. Clavicle
   h. Humerus
5. Help a child who is immobilized by a skeletal condition plan his diet.
6. Give skin care to a child with skeletal traction.

REVIEW QUESTIONS

1. One of the most common causes of death in a child with muscular dystrophy is
   a. renal failure.
   b. osteomyelitis.
   c. cardiac failure.
   d. liver disease.

2. Legg-Calvé-Perthes disease is most often seen in which age group?
   a. 3–9 years
   b. 5–9 years
   c. 3–10 years
   d. 8–12 years

3. Damage to the epiphyseal plate in fractures involving a child can be serious because of
   a. red blood cell production.
   b. calcium storage.
   c. bone growth.
   d. bone healing.

4. A child is referred to a physician after scoliosis screening. The physician plans to defer treatment and watch the child. You know that his curvature must be less than
   a. 10 degrees.
   b. 20 degrees.
   c. 30 degrees.
   d. 40 degrees.

5. A child with suspected scoliosis might have a(n)
   a. prominent clavicle.
   b. expiratory wheeze.
   c. asymmetry of the shoulders.
   d. delayed breast development.

6. Which of the following diseases is usually inherited as an X-linked disorder?
   a. Legg-Calvé-Perthes disease
   b. scoliosis
   c. juvenile rheumatoid arthritis
   d. Duchenne's muscular dystrophy

7. Treatment of Legg-Calvé-Perthes disease consists of
   a. complete bed rest.
   b. no weight-bearing activity.
   c. surgery.
   d. ambulation-abduction casts or braces.

8. Healing of a fracture in a child is
   a. about the same as in an adult.
   b. slower than in an adult.
   c. faster than in an adult.

9. Treatment of osteomyelitis includes the use of
   a. steroids.
   b. antibiotics.
   c. traction.
   d. hydrotherapy.

10. The development of iridocyclitis is a complication of
    a. Legg-Calvé-Perthes disease.
    b. osteomyelitis.
    c. juvenile rheumatoid arthritis.
    d. scoliosis.

11. A liquid that helps to neutralize the alkaline content of the urine and thus decrease the risk of a bladder infection is
    a. coffee.
    b. orange juice.
    c. cranberry juice.
    d. milk.

Student Name ____________________

12. When caring for a child in Bryant traction, the nurse should
    a. remove the weights when bathing.
    b. support the weights when the bed is moved.
    c. position the child so the buttocks touch the bed.
    d. position the child's legs at right angles to the body.

13. A priority nursing diagnosis for an adolescent treated for osteosarcoma is
    a. Risk for Infection.
    b. Post-Trauma Response.
    c. Body Image Disturbance.
    d. Risk for Trauma.

14. Adolescent girls who engage in heavy exercise may experience
    a. migraine headaches.
    b. lower back pain.
    c. amenorrhea.
    d. urinary frequency.

15. Legg-Calvé-Perthes disease affects the
    a. tip of the tibia.
    b. shaft of the fibula.
    c. head of the femur.
    d. patella.

16. Young children and infants with osteomyelitis most likely will indicate where the pain is located by
    a. pointing to the area.
    b. showing decreased voluntary movement of the extremity.
    c. verbalizing the site.
    d. drawing a picture.

17. The mother of an infant born with congenital torticollis is concerned that her child will always have limited neck motion. You know that
    a. the child will always need to wear a neck brace.
    b. surgery is the treatment of choice.
    c. the condition will most probably resolve by two to six months.
    d. there is nothing the mother can do to assist in the resolution of the condition.

18. A child is being removed from the home of an abusive parent. The child is crying and a co-worker wonders if this could be a sign that the child was not abused. You know that
    a. the child would not be crying if they had been abused in the home.
    b. the child will mourn the loss of the family, even if there was abuse.
    c. the child is seeking attention.
    d. the child doesn't really understand what is happening.

19. Which of the following statements by a mother might indicate future problems related to the care of a newborn infant?

    a. "I am happy that my mother will be here for a few weeks. I feel overwhelmed caring for the baby and my other children."

    b. "May I call you with questions? This is my first child and although I feel prepared, I am feeling frightened by the responsibility."

    c. "The baby cries all of the time. She doesn't seem to like me. I didn't think it would be like this. Sometimes I think she is just trying to irritate me."

    d. "Our baby has colic. We are taking turns rocking her and getting up with her at night. When will we get a full night of sleep?"

Student Name ____________________

chapter **25**

The Child with a Respiratory or Cardiovascular Disorder

LEARNING ACTIVITIES

1. Match the terms in the left column with their definitions on the right (a–d).

_____ hypothermia	a. intestines of the infant become obstructed with meconium while *in utero*
_____ meconium ileus	b. reduces the body tissue temperature
_____ polycythemia	c. asthma attack lasting several days
_____ status asthmaticus	d. increased red blood cells

2. List six of the more common procedures used to diagnose respiratory conditions.

   a. ____________________

   b. ____________________

   c. ____________________

   d. ____________________

   e. ____________________

   f. ____________________

3. The common cold is also known as ____________________.

4. List five measures that can relieve the symptoms of the common cold.

   a. ______________________________

   b. ______________________________

   c. ______________________________

   d. ______________________________

   e. ______________________________

5. Define the term *croup*.

   ____

   ____

   ____

6. Describe the clinical course of laryngotracheobronchitis.

   ____

   ____

   ____

   ____

   ____

   ____

7. What advice would you give a parent about home care of a child with croup?

   ____

   ____

   ____

   ____

   ____

8. If epiglottitis is suspected, what nursing responsibility must be instituted?
   ____

9. The treatment of choice for a child with epiglottitis is a ____________________ or ______________________________.

Case Study" Chapter 5 Amy Adams 28 yrs old (WORKbook)

1) Multigravida (had more than on pregnancy)
(2) Primipara (a stillborn birth)
(3) ~~PI~~H (hypertension c̄ two pregnancy)
(4) Gestation pregnant (LGA)

A(2) asking her history of pregnancy.
3.

B. She should be taught how to select appropriate (diet) foods, how to (✓) her blood sugar

C. The nurse must help her to understand the importance of bedrest + to find way to manage it. The nurse must impress how important rest is to her baby's well-being.

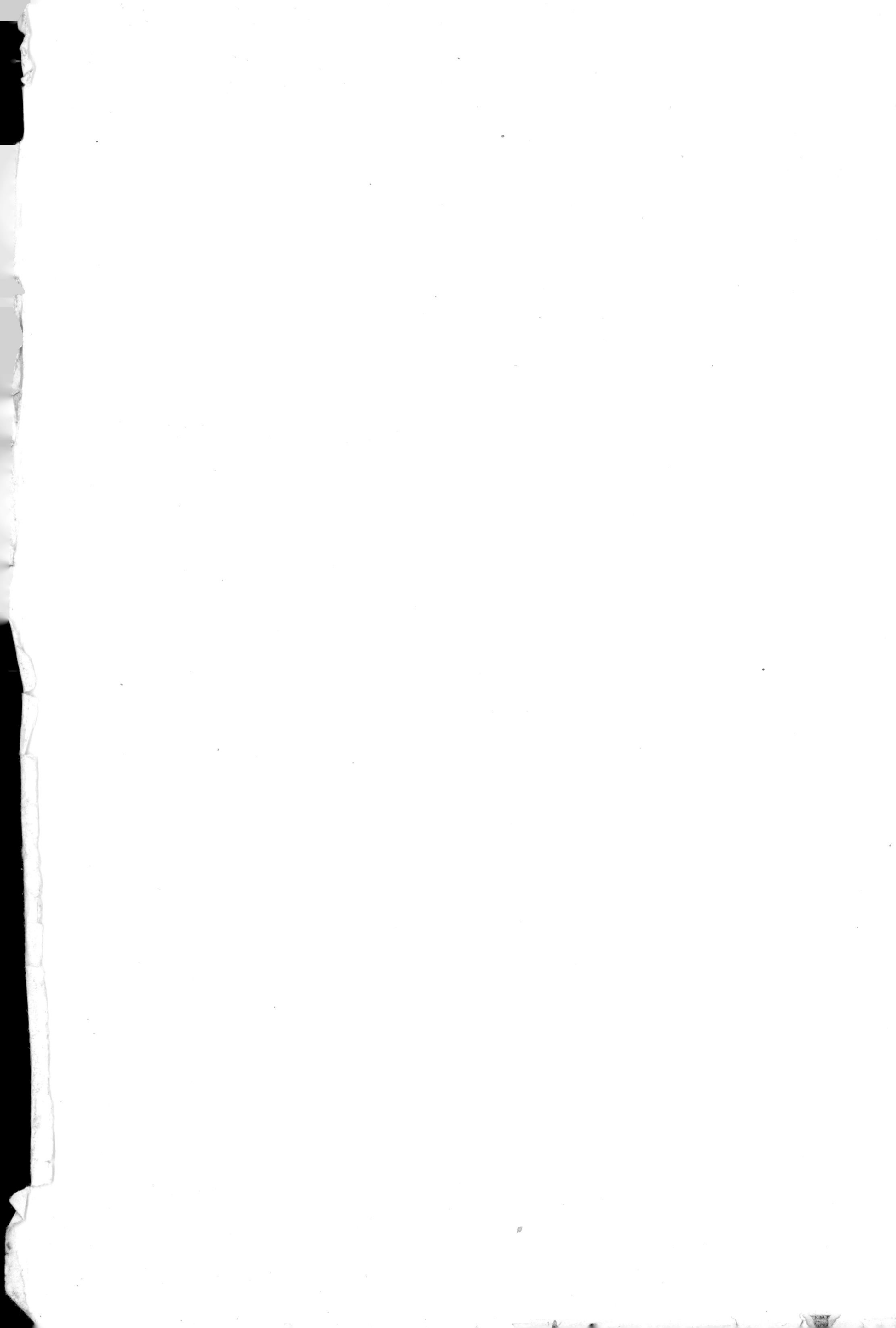

Student Name ______________________________

10. List the common signs and symptoms of bronchiolitis.

    a. ______________________________

    b. ______________________________

    c. ______________________________

    d. ______________________________

11. Respiratory syncytial virus (RSV) is spread by ______________________________.

12. RSV can survive for more than ________ hours on countertops, tissues, and soap.

13. List four reasons why children are at greater risk than adults to develop more severe respiratory infections.

    a. ______________________________

    b. ______________________________

    c. ______________________________

    d. ______________________________

14. Infants breathe more easily when in the ______________________________ position.

15. List four of the possible signs of respiratory distress.

    a. ______________________________

    b. ______________________________

    c. ______________________________

    d. ______________________________

16. What are some of the common signs and symptoms of pneumonia?

    a. ______________________________

    b. ______________________________

    c. ______________________________

    d. ______________________________

17. The removal of the tonsils and adenoids should wait until the child is at least ______________________ years of age.

18. What signs and symptoms are indicative of bleeding in the postoperative tonsillectomy patient?

    a. ______________________________

    b. ______________________________

    c. ______________________________

    d. ______________________________

19. Describe the pathologic changes that take place in asthma.

    ____

    ____

    ____

    ____

    ____

20. List five signs and symptoms of asthma.

    a. ______________________________

    ____

    b. ______________________________

    ____

    c. ______________________________

    ____

    d. ______________________________

    ____

    e. ______________________________

    ____

21. Why should milk products be avoided by asthmatics?

    ____

22. Describe the stools of a child with cystic fibrosis.

    ____

    ____

Student Name ______________________________

23. What physiologic changes take place in the pancreas of a child who has cystic fibrosis?

____

____

____

____

24. The ______________________________ is the test of choice for diagnosing cystic fibrosis.

25. List three ways respiratory complications can be decreased in patients with cystic fibrosis.

    a. ______________________________

    ____

    b. ______________________________

    ____

    c. ______________________________

    ____

26. Discharge teaching of a child with cystic fibrosis should include instructions about

    a. ______________________________

    b. ______________________________

    c. ______________________________

    d. ______________________________

    e. ______________________________

    f. ______________________________

27. Children with cystic fibrosis should receive which vitamin supplements?

____

28. One of the greatest challenges for the family and the child who is technology-dependent is to maintain optimum ______________ and ______________.

29. List three of the possible conditions that could put a mother at risk for bearing a child with a congenital heart defect.

    a. ______________________________

    b. ______________________________

    c. ______________________________

30. ______________________________ are the leading cause of death among the congenital anomalies during the first year of life.

31. Heart defects can be classified as lesions that

    a. ______________________________

    b. ______________________________

    c. ______________________________

32. Match the types of heart defects on the left with their definitions on the right (a–d).

_____ ventricular septal defect	a. narrowing of the aortic arch or the descending aorta
_____ coarctation of the aorta	b. opening between the right and left ventricles
_____ atrial septal defect	c. failure of the ductus arteriosus to close
_____ patent ductus arteriosus	d. opening between left and right atria

33. Why are prophylactic antibiotics given to children with ventricular septal defects?
    ____

34. What is the classic sign of coarctation of the aorta?

    ____

    ____

    ____

35. In a child with an atrial septal defect, you would expect ______________ ______________ blood to move from the ______________ atrium to the ______________ atrium.

Student Name ______________________________

36. List the signs and symptoms of patent ductus arteriosus.

    a. ______________________________

    ____

    b. ______________________________

    ____

    c. ______________________________

    ____

    d. ______________________________

    ____

37. Describe the four defects that make up tetralogy of Fallot.

    a. ______________________________

    b. ______________________________

    c. ______________________________

    d. ______________________________

38. List the signs and symptoms of tetralogy of Fallot.

    a. ______________________________

    b. ______________________________

    c. ______________________________

    d. ______________________________

    e. ______________________________

    f. ______________________________

    g. ______________________________

39. Explain why polycythemia develops in children with heart defects.

    ____

    ____

40. List four signs and symptoms of congestive heart failure.

    a. ____________________

    b. ____________________

    c. ____________________

    d. ____________________

41. Respirations over ________ breaths/minute are significant in a newborn.

42. Nursing goals when caring for a child with a heart defect include

    a. ____________________

    b. ____________________

    c. ____________________

    d. ____________________

    e. ____________________

    f. ____________________

43. List three nursing actions you could take to conserve the energy of a child with a heart defect.

    a. ____________________

    ____

    b. ____________________

    ____

    c. ____________________

    ____

44. Children receiving diuretics must have their serum ____________________ monitored closely.

45. List four foods high in potassium.

    a. ____________________

    b. ____________________

    c. ____________________

    d. ____________________

Student Name ____

46. What advice would you give an adolescent who shows a consistently high blood pressure reading?

____

____

47. List the signs and symptoms of digitalis toxicity.

a. ____

b. ____

c. ____

d. ____

e. ____

48. What are the classic symptoms of rheumatic fever?

a. ____

____

b. ____

____

c. ____

____

49. Rheumatic fever can be avoided by prevention of ______________ and early treatment of ______________________________.

THINKING CRITICALLY

1. Plan for the discharge of a child newly diagnosed with cystic fibrosis. Include diet, medication, respiratory care, and psychologic care of the child and the parents.

2. Plan activities for a child with congestive heart disease. Consider the child's need to conserve energy.

3. Develop a plan of care for a child with a congenital heart defect. Incorporate into the plan the child's physiologic and psychologic needs.

CASE STUDIES

1. Eric, an 18-month-old toddler, is admitted to the hospital with pneumonia and is placed in a Croupette and an IV is started.
    a. Eric's mother is upset because her oldest child died of pneumonia when she was an infant. What should you tell her about the current prognosis of the disease? Support your answer with a rationale.
    b. The physician notes that he will discontinue the IV when the child takes adequate oral fluids. What should you do to encourage this to happen?
    c. Describe the various stages of activity the child will go through as he progresses through the disease. Start with him on bed rest.

2. Six-year-old Jasmine is admitted to the hospital with a diagnosis of asthma. She is restless, has difficulty breathing, and is wheezing. She has numerous allergies.
    a. Jasmine relates that she has been taking allergy shots and they have removed many of the objects she is allergic to from their home. Explain each of these methods of allergy treatment.
    b. What position should Jasmine be in to decrease respiratory distress?
    c. The physician wants Jasmine to have increased oral intake. What liquids should be encouraged and which should be avoided?
    d. Jasmine wants to participate in the swim team at school. What should the nurse tell her about asthma and exercise?

3. Alicia, an eight-year-old child, is admitted to the hospital with cystic fibrosis. She has a history of chronic pulmonary and sinus problems.
    a. Alicia takes an oral pancreatic extract. When should she take this medication?
    b. Alicia has extensive lung disease. What measures would improve respirations?
    c. What type of diet would be ordered for Alicia?
    d. Alicia is anorexic. What can be done to increase her intake?

Student Name ____________________

OTHER LEARNING ACTIVITIES

1. Observe a cardiac catheterization in the clinical area.
2. Care for a child with cardiac disease.
3. Care for a child who has had cardiac surgery.
4. Care for a child in a oxygen tent who has a respiratory disease.
5. Care for a child who has had a tonsillectomy.
6. Admit a child to the unit who has asthma.
7. Teach a child with cystic fibrosis about respiratory care and diet.
8. Become certified in pediatric CPR.
9. While in the clinical area, locate the emergency cart for the unit you are working on.

REVIEW QUESTIONS

1. The most common heart defect in children is
   a. ventricular septal defect.
   b. coarctation of the aorta.
   c. atrial septal defect.
   d. patent ductus arteriosus.

2. The best method of feeding infants with heart defects is to
   a. space feedings at least every three to four hours.
   b. give frequent large feedings.
   c. feed intravenously.
   d. feed on demand.

3. If the pulse of a newborn is below _______ bpm, digitalis is withheld.
   a. 120
   b. 110
   c. 100
   d. 90

4. Signs and symptoms of digitoxin toxicity include
   a. retention of water.
   b. diarrhea.
   c. nausea and vomiting.
   d. headaches.

5. When a child is on diuretics, it is the nurse's responsibility to
   a. withhold fluids.
   b. monitor serum electrolyte levels.
   c. place on seizure precautions.
   d. check the dosage with another nurse before giving.

6. A child who is hypertensive is identified during routine screening. The child should be
   a. placed on diuretics.
   b. placed on beta-adrenergic blockers.
   c. put on an exercise and diet program.
   d. scheduled for two more blood pressure readings.

7. An increase in nasopharyngitis in children would be expected when they
   a. enter preschool.
   b. have a change in their routine.
   c. play outdoors.
   d. enter junior high.

8. An appropriate treatment for a child with bronchiolitis is
   a. isolation.
   b. increased fluids.
   c. antihistamines.
   d. increased solids.

9. The best liquid to give to a child who has had a tonsillectomy is
   a. orange juice.
   b. milk.
   c. hot chocolate.
   d. popsicle.

10. A child who has had a tonsillectomy and adenoidectomy becomes upset and cries when the nurse attempts to apply an ice pack to his throat. The nurse should
    a. restrain him and apply the pack.
    b. sedate him and apply the pack.
    c. remove the pack.
    d. wait until he falls asleep and then apply the pack.

11. A child with cystic fibrosis should be placed on a diet that is
    a. high calorie, high protein, moderate fat.
    b. high calorie, low protein, low fat.
    c. low calorie, high protein, low fat.
    d. high calorie, low protein, moderate fat.

12. Children with croup are placed in an environment of high humidity in order to
    a. decrease the possibility of a bacterial infection.
    b. increase the child's appetite.
    c. liquefy secretions.
    d. decrease body temperature.

13. If a child is suspected of having epiglottitis, the nurse should
    a. avoid examination of the pharynx.
    b. force fluids.
    c. place the child on the right side.
    d. place the child in isolation.

14. Which of the following could indicate a postoperative emergency in a tonsillectomy patient?
    a. sore throat
    b. vomiting pink-tinged blood
    c. low-grade fever
    d. frequent swallowing

15. The child with asthma should be instructed to
    a. avoid exercise.
    b. avoid hot liquids.
    c. identify early signs of an asthma attack.
    d. decrease the amount of liquids taken after 6:00 P.M.

16. A child with a congenital heart abnormality would most likely experience
    a. difficulty feeding.
    b. difficulty sleeping.
    c. normal weight gain.
    d. decreased blood pressure.

Student Name ________________________________

17. Children receiving theophylline may exhibit
    a. decreased pulse.
    b. lethargy.
    c. constipation.
    d. restlessness.

18. Fluids offered to the child with asthma should not be too cold because cold fluids may
    a. increase the chance of dehydration.
    b. trigger reflex bronchospasm.
    c. cause nausea and vomiting.
    d. increase mucus.

19. Children with chronic diseases who are overprotected by their parents
    a. may be more secure.
    b. may have lower self-esteem.
    c. may be more compliant.
    d. may ask more questions.

20. Discharge teaching for the parents of a child with asthma should begin
    a. when a discharge date has been identified.
    b. after the child begins to feel better.
    c. when the parents request information.
    d. on the day of admission.

chapter **26**

The Child with a Condition of the Blood, Blood Forming Organs, or Lymph System

LEARNING ACTIVITIES

1. Match the terms in the left column with their definitions on the right (a–l).

_____ alopecia
_____ ecchymoses
_____ erythrocytes
_____ extramedullary
_____ hemarthrosis
_____ leukocytes
_____ myelosuppression
_____ petechiae
_____ purpura
_____ splenomegaly
_____ thrombocytes

a. groups of adjoining petechiae
b. red blood cells (RBCs)
c. bluish, nonblanching, pinpoint-size lesion
d. white blood cells (WBCs)
e. platelets
f. hemorrhage into a joint cavity
g. depression of normal function of bone marrow
h. enlargement of the spleen
i. loss of hair
j. hemorrhagic spots in the skin, larger than petechiae
k. outside the bone marrow

2. What are the functions of leukocytes and erythrocytes?

____

____

____

____

Student Name ____________________

3. List two common tests performed to determine blood disorders.

   a. ____________________

   b. ____________________

4. List the causes of iron deficiency anemia.

   a. ____________________

   b. ____________________

   c. ____________________

   d. ____________________

5. List four food sources high in iron content.

   a. ____________________

   b. ____________________

   c. ____________________

   d. ____________________

6. List the major signs and symptoms of iron-deficiency anemia.

   a. ____________________

   b. ____________________

   c. ____________________

   d. ____________________

7. Infants should be screened for iron-deficiency anemia at __________ and __________ months of age.

8. Explain the procedure for giving Imferon.

   ____

   ____

   ____

9. Describe the stools of infants on iron supplements.

   ____

10. What should the nurse tell a mother about the type of milk an infant should receive during the first year of life?

   ____

   ____

11. Sickle cell disease is most prevalent in the ______________________________ ______________________________ population.

12. List four factors that might trigger a sickle cell crisis.

    a. ______________________________

    b. ______________________________

    c. ______________________________

    d. ______________________________

13. Explain the difference between sickle cell trait and sickle cell disease.

    ____

    ____

    ____

    ____

14. List three of the possible signs and symptoms of a sickle cell crisis.

    a. ______________________________

    b. ______________________________

    c. ______________________________

15. List four observations you would make when caring for a child in sickle cell crisis.

    a. ______________________________

       ____

    b. ______________________________

       ____

    c. ______________________________

       ____

    d. ______________________________

       ____

16. What is the most common test used to screen for sickle cell disease?

    ____

Student Name ____________________

17. List two priority goals when caring for a child with sickle cell disease.

    a. ____________________

    b. ____________________

18. ____________________ is a nasal spray that can stop bleeding and may be the treatment of choice for mild cases of hemophilia.

19. When bleeding occurs in a child with hemophilia, the traditional approach is to include ____________, ____________, ____________ and ____________.

20. Hemophilia A is inherited as a sex-linked ____________________ trait.

21. The classic clinical manifestation of hemophilia is ____________________.

22. List four nursing interventions appropriate for the child with alopecia.

    a. ____________________

    b. ____________________

    c. ____________________

    d. ____________________

23. Describe the preschooler's response to a sibling's death.

    ____

    ____

    ____

24. A common side effect of radiation is ____________________.

25. The stages of dying according to Kubler-Ross include

    a. ____________________

    b. ____________________

    c. ____________________

    d. ____________________

    e. ____________________

    f. ____________________

26. Following a splenectomy, the child faces the long-term risk of serious ____________.

27. Describe the clinical manifestations of idiopathic thrombocytopenic purpura (ITP).

____

____

____

____

28. A toddler with ITP would have the most difficulty following which part of the treatment? _______________

29. Explain the pathologic changes that take place when a child has leukemia.

____

____

____

30. List seven of the possible presenting signs and symptoms of leukemia.

a. _______________

b. _______________

c. _______________

d. _______________

e. _______________

f. _______________

g. _______________

31. List the five phases of treatment of leukemia.

a. _______________

b. _______________

c. _______________

d. _______________

e. _______________

Student Name ______________________________

32. List some of the common side effects of chemotherapy.

    a. ______________________________

    b. ______________________________

    c. ______________________________

    d. ______________________________

    e. ______________________________

33. What skin care interventions should be given to the adolescent with Hodgkin's disease who has received radiation?

    ____

    ____

34. List the types of sickle cell crises.

    a. ______________________________

    b. ______________________________

    c. ______________________________

    d. ______________________________

THINKING CRITICALLY

1. List four nursing diagnoses and the goals and interventions that would be appropriate for a child in sickle cell crisis.

2. List three nursing diagnoses for a child with leukemia in relation to skin care, mobility, and nutrition. Give the nursing interventions for your diagnoses.

CASE STUDY

1. Lauren, a five-year-old girl, is hospitalized with acute lymphocytic leukemia (ALL). She is receiving chemotherapy and has been placed in a private room.

   a. What special precautions should be taken with a child who is immune-suppressed?

   b. Lauren develops ulcerations in her mouth. What can the nurse do to relieve discomfort and promote healing of the oral mucosa?

   c. Lauren is to receive a unit of packed red blood cells. For what signs and symptoms of a reaction should the nurse observe and what action would be taken if a reaction occurred?

OTHER LEARNING ACTIVITIES

1. While in the clinical area, care for a child who has cancer and is receiving chemotherapy.

2. While in the clinical area, care for a child who is in sickle cell crisis.

3. Observe a bone marrow aspiration being performed.

4. Speak with a pediatric nurse who works with children who have cancer about her feelings when a child dies.

5. Visit the Ronald McDonald House in your city. Discuss with your classmates the setting and the services.

6. Discuss with your classmates your feelings when you must cause discomfort to a child in order to help him/her.

REVIEW QUESTIONS

1. The highest incidence of iron-deficiency anemia occurs in which age group?

   a. infants

   b. toddlers

   c. preschool children

   d. school-age children

2. Iron stores are reduced in

   a. infants who are large for gestational age.

   b. preterm infants.

   c. blond infants.

   d. infants with birth defects.

3. Iron absorption is increased by taking it with

   a. orange juice.

   b. cereal.

   c. milk.

   d. eggs.

4. It is recommended that iron-fortified formula be given to infants through age

   a. 3 months.

   b. 6 months.

   c. 9 months.

   d. 12 months.

Student Name ______________________________

5. Which of the following presents the greatest risk to the child with hemophilia?

    a. hematuria

    b. hemarthrosis

    c. intracranial bleeding

    d. anemia

6. Signs and symptoms that might indicate that a child has idiopathic (immunologic) thrombocytopenic purpura include

    a. headaches and hematuria.

    b. anemia and hemarthrosis.

    c. petechiae and purpura.

    d. hematuria and petechiae.

7. The diagnostic test that confirms a diagnosis of leukemia is a(n)

    a. spinal tap.

    b. bone marrow aspiration.

    c. complete blood count.

    d. x-ray of the bones.

8. When caring for a child on steroid therapy, it is important to seek immediate medical attention if the child

    a. vomits.

    b. develops a fever.

    c. skips a meal.

    d. gains weight.

9. Intake can sometimes be increased in children who have leukemia by

    a. having the parents bring food from home.

    b. pointing out to the child that he will not get well if he doesn't eat.

    c. insisting on a strict eating schedule.

    d. asking the parents to avoid coming to visit during meals.

10. Children with Hodgkin's disease usually present with a(n)

    a. rapid weight loss.

    b. painless cervical neck lump.

    c. enlarged abdomen.

    d. high fever.

11. Children with hemophilia should avoid

    a. swimming.

    b. salicylates.

    c. citrus fruits.

    d. analgesics.

12. Children with sickle cell trait

    a. have a 10% chance of developing the disease.

    b. have a 25% chance of developing the disease.

    c. have a 50% chance of developing the disease.

    d. will not develop the disease.

13. A child admitted to the hospital in sickle cell crisis should

    a. have ice applied to painful areas.

    b. be encouraged to ambulate.

    c. be placed on increased intake and output.

    d. not be given narcotics.

14. Immediate nursing care of a child with hemophilia who has hemarthrosis includes

    a. application of heat.

    b. active and passive range-of-motion exercises.

    c. immobilization of the area.

    d. withholding Factor VIII.

15. The greatest concern of a nurse caring for a child with ITP is
    a. noncompliance with aspirin therapy.
    b. a reaction to platelets.
    c. injuries that might initiate bleeding.
    d. development of a secondary bacterial infection.

16. Anxiety can be decreased in both the family and the child who has cancer by
    a. not telling the child that he/she has cancer.
    b. explaining all procedures before they are done.
    c. placing the child with an older child who has the same diagnosis.
    d. discouraging the child and parents from discussing the issue of death.

17. A common childhood disease that can have devastating effects on an immune-suppressed child is
    a. measles.
    b. chickenpox.
    c. rubella.
    d. nasopharyngitis.

18. Nursing care of an adolescent with cancer who is refusing to cooperate with treatment should include
    a. asking the parents to make the adolescent cooperate.
    b. allowing the adolescent to make some choices.
    c. withholding favorite foods until the behavior changes.
    d. restricting visitors until the behavior is modified.

19. The risk for damage to the kidney during treatment for cancer can be decreased by
    a. drinking cranberry juice.
    b. forcing fluids.
    c. taking anticoagulants.
    d. drinking hot tea.

20. A child with cancer refuses mouth care. The best response is
    a. "We can wait until the next time when you are not so uncomfortable."
    b. "I will see if the doctor will let us stop doing mouth care."
    c. "If you will cooperate this time, we can skip mouth care later today."
    d. "Although I know it is uncomfortable, we must do this to prevent even more problems in your mouth."

Student Name ______________________________

chapter **27**

The Child with a Gastrointestinal Condition

LEARNING ACTIVITIES

1. Match the terms in the left column with their definitions on the right (a–i).

_____ homeostasis	a. protrusion of part of the intestine through the umbilical ring
_____ hyperpnea	b. constricted hernia
_____ incarcerated	c. protrusion of part of the abdominal contents through the inguinal canal
_____ inguinal hernia	d. the eating of nonfood items
_____ pica	e. operation to correct pyloric stenosis
_____ projectile vomiting	f. state of equilibrium of the body
_____ pyloromyotomy	g. narrowing
_____ stenosis	h. vomiting in which the stomach contents are forcibly ejected
_____ umbilical hernia	i. increased respiratory rate

2. List four of the possible common tests used to diagnose gastrointestinal disorders.

   a. ______________________________

   b. ______________________________

   c. ______________________________

   d. ______________________________

3. The infant with tracheo-esophageal fistula will ______________________ and ______________________ when the first feeding is given.

4. Gluten is found in ______________, ______________, ______________, and ______________________.

5. Stools in the child with celiac disease are ________________, ______________, and ________________________________.

6. Surgical repair of a hernia is called a ____.

7. Describe the usual progression of signs and symptoms in a child with pyloric stenosis.

____

____

____

____

8. A complication of the vomiting associated with pyloric stenosis is ______________________________________.

9. Describe the progression of feeding after postoperative correction of pyloric stenosis.

____

____

____

____

____

10. Describe the initial onset of intussusception.

____

____

____

____

11. Treatment of choice of intussusception is reduction through the use of a ____.

12. To prevent aspiration of vomitus after feeding, a child should be placed in what position?

____

Student Name ____________________

13. What are the priorities of documentation for a child who is vomiting?

    a. ____________________

    b. ____________________

    c. ____________________

    d. ____________________

    e. ____________________

    f. ____________________

    g. ____________________

14. ____________________ is the greatest threat to life in isotonic dehydration.

15. Nursing interventions related to gastroenteritis focus on

    a. ____________________

    b. ____________________

    c. ____________________

16. The earliest sign of Hirschsprung's disease is failure to pass meconium stools within ________ to ________ hours after birth.

17. Teaching parents about prevention of gastroenteritis includes

    a. ____________________

    b. ____________________

    c. ____________________

    d. ____________________

18. The child with gastroesophageal reflux disease should be placed in which position after feeding? ____________________.

19. Tap water enemas are never given to children because they can lead to ____________________ and ____________________.

20. Failure to thrive (FTT) describes infants and children who:

____

____

____

____

21. List four sources of lead poisoning.

a. _______________

b. _______________

c. _______________

d. _______________

22. List four of the possible common signs and symptoms seen in the early stages of lead poisoning.

a. _______________

b. _______________

c. _______________

d. _______________

23. Describe the treatment of lead poisoning.

____

____

____

____

24. Activated charcoal should not be given with _______________ because it will neutralize both, rendering both ineffective in the treatment of poisoning.

25. How is nystatin applied to the mouth of a child with thrush?

____

Student Name ______________________________

26. The goals in the treatment of poisoning are

    a. ______________________________

    b. ______________________________

    c. ______________________________

    d. ______________________________

27. Ipecac should not be used with ______________________________, or ______________________________.

28. List three foods that may be given to the older child with diarrhea.

    a. ______________________________

    b. ______________________________

    c. ______________________________

29. Signs and symptoms of dehydration in the infant include

    a. ______________________________

    b. ______________________________

    c. ______________________________

    d. ______________________________

30. Explain how pinworm infestation is spread.

    ____

    ____

    ____

    ____

31. What is the most common sign of pinworms?

    ____

32. Describe the treatment of pinworms.

____

____

____

____

____

____

____

33. List five typical signs and symptoms of kwashiorkor.

a. ____

b. ____

c. ____

d. ____

e. ____

34. List three signs and symptoms of rickets.

a. ____

b. ____

c. ____

35. The decrease of incidence of rickets in the world is attributed to ______________________.

THINKING CRITICALLY

1. You are caring for a child who drank a poisonous substance. How can you assist the parents? What feelings might they be having?

Student Name ____________________

CASE STUDY

1. Six-month-old Amber is diagnosed as failing to thrive. Amber's mother is a single parent who does not work outside the home. Neighbors report that they often hear Amber crying and that her mother seldom holds her. They also report that Amber's mother has related to them that being a mother is not what she thought it would be.
   a. List some of the signs of failure to thrive.
   b. What treatment might be implemented?
   c. How would you involve Amber's mother in her care?
   d. Discuss your feelings towards parents who neglect their children.

OTHER LEARNING ACTIVITIES

1. Observe an endoscopy.
2. Use Figure 27-1 in the textbook to label the following.
   a. Esophagus
   b. Stomach
   c. Pancreas
   d. Liver
   e. Gallbladder
   f. Small intestine
   g. Large intestine
   h. Rectum
3. Develop a teaching plan related to poison prevention.
4. Develop a teaching plan related to caring for a child with diarrhea.

REVIEW QUESTIONS

1. The upper GI tract can be visualized through
   a. colonoscopy.
   b. sigmoidoscopy.
   c. endoscopy.
   d. proctoscopy.
2. Children with failure to thrive fall below the ________ percentile on growth charts.
   a. 3rd
   b. 6th
   c. 10th
   d. 15th

3. Which approach might best support maternal attachment when caring for a child with failure to thrive?

   a. Point out areas where the mother needs improvement.

   b. Send the mother to a parenting class.

   c. Role-model appropriate care of the child.

   d. Leave the room when the mother visits.

4. Signs and symptoms of pinworms are

   a. diarrhea, itching, and fever.

   b. nausea, vomiting, and itching.

   c. nausea, vomiting, and weight loss.

   d. itching, irritability, and restlessness.

5. Children with intussusception may have bowel movements containing blood and mucus and no feces. These are called

   a. currant-jelly stools.

   b. mucoid stools.

   c. steatorrhea.

   d. occult blood stools.

6. A newborn's total body weight is about _____ water.

   a. 77%

   b. 65%

   c. 55%

   d. 45%

7. Before potassium is added to an IV, the nurse should

   a. take a baseline blood pressure.

   b. darken the room.

   c. establish that the child is voiding.

   d. place the child on a cardiac monitor.

8. Persistent vomiting can lead to

   a. acidosis.

   b. alkalosis.

   c. hyperkalemia.

   d. hypervolemia.

9. The greatest threat to life in isotonic dehydration is

   a. hypervolemic shock.

   b. hypovolemic shock.

   c. respiratory acidosis.

   d. respiratory alkalosis.

10. A classic sign of pyloric stenosis is

   a. constipation.

   b. projectile vomiting.

   c. diarrhea.

   d. anorexia.

11. When a child has pinworms, the nurse knows that

   a. it is a sign of poor hygiene.

   b. the child will be hospitalized.

   c. all family members should be treated.

   d. a warm stool specimen is sent to the lab.

12. Most umbilical hernias

   a. disappear by one year of age.

   b. must be repaired at birth.

   c. can be reduced by taping the area.

   d. are repaired by two years of age.

Student Name ______________________________

13. Treatment of gastroesophageal reflux disease includes
    a. feeding half-strength formula.
    b. positioning in an infant seat after feeding.
    c. increasing the time between feedings.
    d. placing the infant prone with the head elevated after feeding.

14. The earliest sign of Hirschsprung's disease is
    a. failure to pass meconium stools.
    b. chronic constipation of the newborn.
    c. chronic diarrhea of the newborn.
    d. ribbon-like stools.

15. Children who are receiving treatment for lead poisoning should be involved in
    a. physical therapy.
    b. syringe play.
    c. psychotherapy.
    d. support groups.

16. The organ damaged by acetaminophen poisoning is the
    a. gallbladder.
    b. pancreas.
    c. liver.
    d. stomach.

17. One aspect of treatment of the child with pinworms is to
    a. place the family on antibiotics.
    b. isolate the child from the rest of the family.
    c. wash the bed linens in hot water.
    d. monitor the child's temperature.

18. Preoperative care of the child with Hirschsprung's disease may include
    a. tap water enemas.
    b. frequent rectal temperatures.
    c. taking axillary temperatures
    d. administration of laxatives.

19. Infants are more susceptible to accidental ingestion of nonfood objects because
    a. they are often left unattended.
    b. they are curious.
    c. they are constantly hungry.
    d. they want the attention.

20. The infant who is NPO prior to having a pyloromyotomy for pyloric stenosis can have his/her sucking needs met through
    a. occasional sips of water.
    b. providing a straw for sucking.
    c. providing a pacifier.
    d. sucking on a wet washcloth.

chapter **28**

The Child with a Genitourinary Condition

LEARNING ACTIVITIES

1. Match the terms in the left column with their definitions on the right (a–k).

_____ cystitis
_____ encopresis
_____ enuresis
_____ glomeruli
_____ hypospadias
_____ neutropenia
_____ phimosis
_____ pyelonephritis
_____ urgency
_____ urethritis
_____ vesicoureteral reflux

a. backward flow of urine into the ureters
b. abnormal number of voidings in a short period of time
c. inflammation of the bladder
d. infection of the kidney substance and pelvis
e. infection of the ureters
f. uncontrolled voiding after bladder control has been established
g. narrowing of the preputial opening of the foreskin
h. the working units of the kidney
i. abnormally low levels of granulocytes
j. congenital defect in which the urinary meatus is not at the end of the penis but on the lower shaft
k. fecal soiling beyond four years of age

Student Name ____

2. The functional unit of the kidney is the ____________________.

3. List six tests used to determine the cause of urinary dysfunction.

   a. ____

   b. ____

   c. ____

   d. ____

   e. ____

   f. ____

4. List four of the possible reasons why urinary tract infections are more common in girls than in boys.

   a. ____

   b. ____

   c. ____

   d. ____

5. Compare the signs and symptoms of a urinary tract infection in infants with those in older children.

	Infant	*Older Child*
a.	____________________	____________________
b.	____________________	____________________
c.	____________________	____________________
d.	____________________	____________________
e.	____________________	____________________
f.	____________________	____________________

6. The characteristic sign of nephrosis is ____________________.

7. Edema associated with nephrosis usually occurs first around the ____________________ and ____________________.

8. What is the treatment of choice for nephrosis?

   ____

9. List three types of skin care that might be given to a child with nephrosis.

   a. ______________________________

   b. ______________________________

   c. ______________________________

10. List three nursing interventions used with a child who is anorexic secondary to nephrosis.

    a. ______________________________

    b. ______________________________

    c. ______________________________

11. When observing the urine of a child with nephrosis, the nurse should note

    a. ______________________________

    b. ______________________________

    c. ______________________________

    d. ______________________________

12. Acute glomerulonephritis is thought to be a(n) ______________________________ ______________________________ reaction caused by ______________________________ ______________________________.

13. List four nursing interventions that would be appropriate for the child who has acute glomerulonephritis.

    a. ______________________________

    b. ______________________________

    c. ______________________________

    d. ______________________________

14. What is involved in the treatment of Wilm's tumor?

    a. ______________________________

    b. ______________________________

    c. ______________________________

Student Name ______________________________

15. What precaution is taken in a child with a Wilm's tumor to prevent spread of the disease?

____

____

16. Surgery for hypospadias is usually performed before age __________ months.

17. What is the rationale for instructing females to wipe their perineal area from front to back? ______________________________

THINKING CRITICALLY

1. A child you are caring for is in renal failure. She is being evaluated for a kidney transplant. Use the library to research this topic. Include in your information the selection process, procedure, risks, expense, recovery, and maintenance.

CASE STUDY

1. A three-year-old child, Tucker, is hospitalized with nephrosis. Tucker is pale, lethargic, anorexic, and has generalized edema.
   a. Tucker is put on steroid therapy. What are three nursing interventions associated with his treatment?
   b. Plan a menu for Tucker for one day using the nutritional requirements necessary for his recovery.
   c. Tucker likes to lie on his stomach. When you change his position, he is irritable and his mother objects. What would you tell his mother?

OTHER LEARNING ACTIVITIES

1. While in the clinical area, collect a urine specimen from an infant and a toddler.
2. Measure abdominal girth on a child with ascites.
3. Keep an intake and output record on a child with kidney disease.
4. Use Figure 28-1 in the textbook to label the following.
   a. Kidney
   b. Ureter
   c. Urinary bladder
   d. Urethra

REVIEW QUESTIONS

1. The treatment of choice for nephrotic syndrome is
   a. diuretics.
   b. antibiotics.
   c. analgesics.
   d. steroids.

2. The child with nephrotic syndrome is at risk for developing
   a. skin breakdown.
   b. an antigen–antibody reaction.
   c. pathologic fractures.
   d. urinary stasis.

3. Children who are immune-suppressed should not
   a. receive antihistamines.
   b. swim.
   c. be immunized.
   d. attend school.

4. What activity restrictions are placed on the child with acute glomerulonephritis?
   a. none
   b. bed rest for two weeks
   c. limited until gross hematuria subsides
   d. limited for two weeks

5. Children with acute glomerulonephritis can develop
   a. chronic urinary stasis.
   b. petechiae.
   c. hypotension.
   d. hypertension.

6. Wilm's tumors are often discovered when
   a. children enter school.
   b. the child has flank pain.
   c. blood is noted in the urine.
   d. a routine physical is given.

7. Which of the following terms describes a urethral opening that is located on the undersurface of the penis?
   a. hydrocele
   b. phimosis
   c. hypospadias
   d. epispadias

8. The risk of urinary tract infections in girls can be lessened by teaching them to
   a. wear nylon underwear.
   b. void only when their bladder is full.
   c. limit fluids after 8:00 P.M.
   d. wipe themselves from the front to the back.

9. When caring for a child with nephrosis, the nurse would expect to do which of these interventions?
   a. weigh weekly
   b. intake and output
   c. force fluids
   d. encourage ambulation

10. Acute glomerulonephritis is thought to be a(n)
    a. antigen–antibody reaction.
    b. autoimmune disease.
    c. primary disease.
    d. infectious disease.

Student Name ______________________________

11. The urine in acute glomerulonephritis can be described as
    a. straw-colored.
    b. smoky brown.
    c. cloudy and concentrated.
    d. yellow with many mucous shreds.

12. A sign of urinary infection in the infant is
    a. weight loss.
    b. abdominal pain.
    c. hematuria.
    d. pain during micturition.

13. You are caring for a child who has a ureterostomy. You can expect
    a. urine to be drained from the pelvis of the kidney.
    b. an opening into the bladder between the umbilicus and pubis.
    c. surgical implantation of ureters to outside the abdominal wall.
    d. a tube above the pubis into the bladder to provide urinary drainage.

14. The nurse should observe the child with an acute urinary tract infection for changes in
    a. pulse, respiration, and temperature.
    b. skin color, respiration, and temperature.
    c. blood pressure, weight, and temperature.
    d. weight, respiration, and pulse.

15. Children receiving steroids should
    a. be placed on antibiotics before there are signs of an infection.
    b. be isolated.
    c. be watched closely for signs of infection.
    d. taken off the medication after one week.

16. When giving skin care to a child with nephrotic syndrome, the nurse should pay special attention to the
    a. mouth, nose, and anus.
    b. neck, axilla, and groin.
    c. genitals, feet, and hands.
    d. axilla, mouth, and hands.

17. When weighing diapers on a gram scale, the conversion from grams to milliliters is
    a. 1 g = 2.5 ml.
    b. 1 g = 1 ml.
    c. 1 g = .5 ml.
    d. 1 g = .25 ml.

18. While the child with nephrotic syndrome is being treated, he/she should not receive
    a. antihistamines.
    b. immunizations.
    c. diuretics.
    d. analgesics.

19. While caring for a child with glomerulonephritis, the nurse observes a rise in the child's blood pressure. The nurse should
    a. document the change.
    b. document and recheck the blood pressure in two hours.
    c. notify the physician.
    d. withhold fluids until the physician can visit.

20. Fruits that acidify urine and therefore decrease the rate of bacterial multiplication include

    a. peaches and strawberries.

    b. cranberries and plums.

    c. bananas and oranges.

    d. pears and prunes.

Student Name ______________________________

chapter **29**

The Child with a Skin Condition

LEARNING ACTIVITIES

1. Match the terms in the left column with their definitions on the right (a–j).

_____ autograft
_____ comedone
_____ debridement
_____ heterograft
_____ homograft
_____ isograft
_____ macule
_____ MRSA
_____ pediculosis
_____ strawberry nevus

a. *Staphylococcus* resistant to antibiotics in current use
b. graft tissue from a source other than human
c. removal of dried crusts
d. graft tissue from cadavers
e. graft tissue from another part of one's body
f. plug of keratin, sebum, and bacteria
g. benign hemangioma that disappears without treatment
h. graft from the patient's identical twin
i. infestation of humans by lice
j. flat rash (freckles)

2. Describe vernix caseosa.

____

____

3. What is the purpose of vernix caseosa?

____

____

4. Name three tests used in diagnosing skin conditions.

   a. ______________________________

   b. ______________________________

   c. ______________________________

5. Name three of the possible characteristics of skin lesions.

   a. ______________________________

   b. ______________________________

   c. ______________________________

6. What is impetigo and how can it be prevented?

   ____

   ____

   ____

7. Describe the treatment of impetigo.

   ____

   ____

   ____

8. How can the nurse support the parents of a child with strawberry nevus?

   ____

   ____

   ____

9. Briefly describe the pathology of acne.

   ____

   ____

10. Patients taking vitamin A should avoid ______________________.

11. The main concern of anyone taking Accutane is to
    ______________________________.

12. Eczema is indicative of ______________________________.

Student Name ______________________________

13. Allergens enter the body of the child with eczema through

 a. ______________________________

 b. ______________________________

 c. ______________________________

 d. ______________________________

14. Describe the application of ointment to the skin of a child with eczema.

____

____

____

15. Name the types and locations of the three kinds of pediculosis.

 a. ______________________________

 b. ______________________________

 c. ______________________________

16. Name the types and locations of the three kinds of tinea fungal infections.

 a. ______________________________

 b. ______________________________

 c. ______________________________

17. Indications of an inhalation problem in a patient who has been burned include

 a. ______________________________

 b. ______________________________

 c. ______________________________

 d. ______________________________

18. If eschar from burns on the trunk inhibits respirations, an ________________ is made in order to prevent restriction of chest movement.

19. Urine output is observed ______________________ in a burn patient.

20. What is the rationale for inserting a nasogastric tube into a burn patient?

21. Describe how a burn wound is dressed.

22. Describe how protective isolation is instituted with a burn patient.

23. List the signs and symptoms of infection in a burn patient.

    a.

    b.

    c.

    d.

    e.

24. What type of diet should a burn patient be given?

    Give an example of a breakfast for an eight-year-old burn patient that would provide the needed nutrients.

Student Name ______________________________

25. List four comfort measures that should be used for the burn patient.

    a. ______________________________

    b. ______________________________

    c. ______________________________

    d. ______________________________

THINKING CRITICALLY

1. Use the nursing process to prepare care for a nine-year-old child who was admitted to the hospital with full-thickness burns of the chest and arms two days ago. He is burned over 15% of his body. His treatment plan includes an IV, reverse isolation, occlusive dressings with Silvadene to the wound, regular diet with high-protein feedings between meals, and morphine for pain. What are the four most important nursing diagnoses? Give the goals of care and nursing interventions for each.

CASE STUDIES

1. Stacey, a 17-year-old teenager diagnosed with acne vulgaris, is prescribed Accutane because other medications have not been effective.

    a. What can the nurse tell Stacey about the side effects of Accutane?

    b. Stacey asks if there is anything she can do with her diet to improve the acne. What should the nurse tell her?

    c. What are some topical preparations that could be recommended for Stacey's acne?

2. Ten-month-old Taylor is admitted to the hospital with a diagnosis of atopic dermatitis. His face, arms, and legs are erythematous and are covered with vesicles, some of which have crusted over. The physician's orders are Isomil formula, continuous wet compresses of Burrow solution to extremities, cut fingernails, and place in private room.

    a. What is infantile eczema (atopic dermatitis)?

    b. What does the order for Isomil have to do with Taylor's diagnosis?

    c. Describe how the nurse will prepare the wet compresses, their purpose, documentation, and any special care that will be taken while they are on Taylor.

    d. What are some of the psychologic needs of a child with eczema?

    e. Taylor is irritable and continually attempts to scratch his arms and legs. What can the nurse do to soothe him?

OTHER LEARNING ACTIVITIES

1. Locate the following on Figure 29-1 in the textbook.
   a. Epidermis
   b. Subcutaneous
   c. Dermis
   d. Blood vessels
   e. Nerve

2. When you are in the clinical setting, read the charts and find a description of skin on
   a. an admission assessment
   b. a child with a skin disorder
   c. a child with a burn

REVIEW QUESTIONS

1. Which of the following is *not* contagious?
   a. impetigo
   b. *Staphylococcus aureus* infection
   c. infantile eczema
   d. pediculosis

2. Treatment of pediculosis capitis includes
   a. treatment of all family members.
   b. washing the hair with hydrogen peroxide.
   c. laundering clothing and bedding in hot water.
   d. cutting the hair of all infested children.

3. First-aid treatment of a partial thickness burn should include
   a. application of butter.
   b. immersion in cold water.
   c. elevation of the involved area.
   d. breaking the blisters.

4. A full thickness burn can best be described as
   a. red with good refill, painful.
   b. mottled, red, dull white, painful.
   c. blistered, pink or red, painful.
   d. tough, leathery, painless to touch.

5. An early sign of sepsis in a burn patient is
   a. decreased pulse.
   b. erythema.
   c. elevated temperature.
   d. decreased blood pressure.

6. A burn patient with cyanosis and charred lips may need a(n)
   a. nasogastric tube.
   b. endotracheal tube.
   c. Foley catheter.
   d. throat culture.

Student Name ____________________

7. Nursing care prior to a dressing change should include
   a. irrigation of nasogastric tube.
   b. administration of pain medication as ordered.
   c. forcing of fluids.
   d. taking the temperature.

8. The priority goal in the management of a severe burn is
   a. wound debridement.
   b. pain control.
   c. fluid replacement.
   d. airway maintenance.

9. A complication of impetigo is
   a. rheumatoid arthritis.
   b. nephritis.
   c. endocarditis.
   d. otitis media.

10. Adolescents on Accutane must
    a. increase their fluid intake.
    b. avoid milk products.
    c. avoid pregnancy.
    d. avoid strenuous exercise.

11. When inspecting children for pediculosis capitis, special attention should be paid to the
    a. pubic area.
    b. hairline at the back of the neck.
    c. area around the forehead.
    d. underarms.

12. A common manifestation of an allergy in a neonate is
    a. asthma.
    b. atopic eczema.
    c. urticaria.
    d. chronic bronchitis.

13. Adolescents with acne should be instructed to
    a. restrict themselves from chocolate and peanuts.
    b. wash their faces at least four times a day.
    c. get adequate rest and eat a well-balanced diet.
    d. avoid sunshine even if they are not on medication.

14. Treatment for eczema includes
    a. not holding the infant.
    b. hot, steaming baths.
    c. dressing the infant warmly.
    d. having wet compresses applied.

15. If the eyebrows and eyelashes are affected by lice, the treatment includes
    a. applying a thick coating of petroleum jelly.
    b. washing with warm, soapy water.
    c. shaving the eyebrows.
    d. applying a prescription shampoo.

16. A priority in changing the dressing of a burn patient is
    a. asking the parents to leave the room.
    b. medicating for pain prior to the procedure.
    c. limiting the number of dressing changes.
    d. doing the procedure in the child's room.

17. A child who has been burned eats only a small amount of the food on her tray. The nurse should
    a. request an order to start an IV.
    b. insert a nasogastric tube for feeding.
    c. offer the child small, frequent feedings.
    d. leave the tray at the bedside longer.

18. A child who was severely burned does not want to leave the hospital. The nurse understands that the child most likely
    a. is a poor student and does not want to return to school.
    b. has grown attached to the staff at the hospital.
    c. is unsure of how others will accept his body changes.
    d. is afraid he will be burned again.

19. Tinea corporis is
    a. usually seen on the soles of the feet.
    b. sometimes transmitted by pets.
    c. treated with a medicated powder.
    d. uncommon in children.

20. Scabies are characterized by
    a. round, dry patches on the arms.
    b. intense itching.
    c. a purulent drainage.
    d. round lesions similar to chickenpox.

Student Name ______________________________

chapter **30**

The Child with a Metabolic Condition

LEARNING ACTIVITIES

1. Match the terms in the left column with their definitions on the right (a–f).

_____ glycosuria	a. excessive thirst
_____ hyperglycemia	b. constant hunger
_____ hypoglycemia	c. increased glucose in the blood
_____ Kussmaul respirations	d. glucose in the urine
_____ polydipsia	e. type of respirations seen in diabetic acidosis
_____ polyphagia	f. decreased glucose in the blood

2. Describe the pathophysiology of diabetes mellitus.

____

____

____

____

3. Explain why diabetes mellitus is more severe in children than adults.

a. ______________________________

b. ______________________________

c. ______________________________

d. ______________________________

4. The onset of insulin-dependent diabetes is increased in pubescent children. Give two possible causes of this increase.

   a. ______________________________

   ____

   b. ______________________________

   ____

5. What are the three "Ps" of insulin-dependent diabetes mellitus (IDDM)?

   a. ______________________________

   b. ______________________________

   c. ______________________________

6. What is the most reliable test to diagnose diabetes mellitus?

   ____

7. What test measures glycemic levels over a period of months?

   ____

8. List the three goals of treatment in IDDM.

   a. ______________________________

   b. ______________________________

   c. ______________________________

9. Children with diabetes have problems associated with their stage of growth and development. Give at least one example of a problem for each age group.

   a. Infant______________________________

   b. Toddler______________________________

   c. Preschool child______________________________

   ____

   d. School-age child______________________________

   ____

   e. Adolescent______________________________

Student Name ______________________________

10. List three goals of nutritional management for the child with IDDM.

    a. ______________________________

    ____

    b. ______________________________

    ____

    c. ______________________________

    ____

11. The standard form of insulin is ___________.

12. Describe insulin injection site rotation.

    ____

    ____

    ____

    ____

    ____

13. List three reasons why a child might go into insulin shock.

    a. ______________________________

    b. ______________________________

    c. ______________________________

14. What is the immediate treatment of a child suspected of having an insulin reaction?

    ____

    ____

15. ______________________________ may be given for the treatment of severe hypoglycemia.

16. Explain the Somogyi phenomenon.

    ____

    ____

    ____

17. List three precautions in the foot care of a child with diabetes.

    a. ______________________________

    b. ______________________________

    ____

    c. ______________________________

    ____

18. When should a child with diabetes check his/her urine for glucose?

    ____

    ____

19. When a child with diabetes plans to travel, what should be done prior to and during the trip?

    a. ______________________________

    b. ______________________________

    c. ______________________________

    ____

    d. ______________________________

20. What is the key treatment of congenital hypothyroidism?

    ____

THINKING CRITICALLY

1. Plot a curve showing the peaks and duration of action for a child who is receiving a combination of regular and NPH insulin at 7:30 A.M. and 5:30 P.M.

CASE STUDY

1. Anne, a 16-year-old teenager, is a newly diagnosed with IDDM. She is a cheerleader and plays basketball. Her parents are constantly with Anne and are very protective of her.

    a. Anne is placed on a constant carbohydrate diet. What should the nurse tell her about the advantages of this type of diet?

    b. Anne asks if she can still play basketball and remain a cheerleader. What should the nurse tell her about these activities?

    c. Anne becomes very impatient with her mother and accuses her of hovering. Can emotional turmoil have an effect on the diabetic?

Student Name ____________________

OTHER LEARNING ACTIVITIES

1. While in the clinical area, teach a child or a parent to give insulin.
2. While in the clinical area, teach a family home glucose monitoring.
3. Care for a child in diabetic ketoacidosis.

REVIEW QUESTIONS

1. Children who receive regular insulin before meals must eat their meal
   a. immediately.
   b. within 15 minutes.
   c. within 40 minutes.
   d. within 60 minutes.

2. Children can usually give their own insulin injections after the age of
   a. 7 years.
   b. 9 years.
   c. 11 years.
   d. 13 years.

3. Children are more prone to insulin reactions than adults because
   a. they tend to have lower blood sugars.
   b. their activities are more irregular.
   c. they take higher doses of insulin.
   d. their metabolism is slower.

4. To treat a child having an insulin reaction, the nurse should give
   a. orange juice.
   b. unsalted crackers.
   c. tea.
   d. an apple.

5. A sign of diabetic ketoacidosis is
   a. cold perspiration.
   b. decreased appetite.
   c. increased thirst.
   d. slurred speech.

6. The most common concentration of insulin is
   a. U-35 insulin.
   b. U-40 insulin.
   c. U-80 insulin.
   d. U-100 insulin.

7. An intermediate type of insulin is
   a. regular insulin.
   b. Lente insulin.
   c. PZI insulin.
   d. ultralente insulin.

8. A frequent cause of hypoglycemia in children is
   a. not enough food.
   b. too much insulin.
   c. illness.
   d. poorly planned exercise.

9. One sign of an insulin reaction is
   a. dry skin.
   b. flushed face.
   c. cold perspiration.
   d. increased thirst.

10. Regular insulin is considered to be a(n)
    a. rapid-acting insulin.
    b. intermediate-acting insulin.
    c. long-acting insulin.

11. A characteristic common to IDDM is that it
    a. is more common in preschool-age children.
    b. is often seen in obese individuals.
    c. always requires insulin.
    d. has few blood sugar fluctuations.

12. One characteristic of Tay-Sachs disease is
    a. diagnosis at birth.
    b. there is no cure.
    c. increased cure rate if diagnosed before age six months.
    d. normal growth and development.

13. Urine should be checked for acetone when the diabetic child
    a. is exercising.
    b. is ill.
    c. has eaten a high-carbohydrate diet.
    d. is going through a growth spurt.

14. Screening infants for hypothyroidism
    a. is ordered for children of high-risk families.
    b. is done on all infants at six months of age.
    c. is done on all infants at birth.
    d. is ineffective.

15. Thyroid hormone replacement for children with hypothyroidism
    a. can be discontinued after the child has gone through puberty.
    b. is lifelong.
    c. is gradually discontinued after the child can eat solids.
    d. is started after the infant is weaned.

Student Name ____________________

chapter **31**

Common Childhood Communicable Diseases

LEARNING ACTIVITIES

1. Match the terms in the left column with their definitions on the right (a–f).

_____ carrier

_____ erythema

_____ fomite

_____ prodromal period

_____ vector

_____ vesicle

a. interval between the earliest symptoms and the appearance of the rash or fever

b. inanimate material that absorbs and transmits infection

c. insect or animal that carries and spreads a disease

d. person who is capable of spreading disease but does not show evidence of it

e. diffused, reddened area on the skin

f. circular, reddened area on the skin that is elevated and contains fluid

2. List three factors related to host resistance to disease.

a. ____________________

b. ____________________

c. ____________________

3. Describe the components of standard precautions.

____

____

____

____

4. Describe the components of protective isolation.

____

____

____

5. List six contraindications to administration of a live virus vaccine.

a. ____

b. ____

c. ____

d. ____

e. ____

f. ____

6. List the common manifestations of chickenpox (varicella).

a. ____

b. ____

c. ____

d. ____

e. ____

f. ____

7. The vaccine given to immunosuppressed children who are exposed to chickenpox is ____.

8. Describe the appearance of the child with fifth disease.
____.

9. List the manifestations of infectious mononucleosis.

a. ____

b. ____

c. ____

d. ____

Student Name ____________________

10. Nursing interventions related to the care of a child with hepatitis A include

    a. ____________________

    b. ____________________

    c. ____________________

    d. ____________________

11. Lyme disease is spread by ____________________.

12. What is the causative agent of AIDS?

    ____

13. List three ways of reducing the risk of contracting STDs.

    a. ____________________

    b. ____________________

    c. ____________________

    d. ____________________

THINKING CRITICALLY

1. You are asked to care for an adolescent with pelvic inflammatory disease. You know that she has been sexually active and has a history of STDs. Think about this situation and then write down your thoughts about this patient.

2. Develop a plan to teach adolescents sex education and the prevention of sexually transmitted diseases.

3. You are caring for a child in isolation. The parents refuse to wear gowns and masks when in the room. What should you do?

OTHER LEARNING ACTIVITIES

1. Contact your local health department for information about educating the public about STDs. Request pamphlets and other written materials.

2. Assist nurses in a public health clinic to administer immunizations.

REVIEW QUESTIONS

1. Which of the following diseases does not require a routine immunization?
   a. chickenpox
   b. smallpox
   c. measles
   d. German measles

2. The period that refers to the initial stage of a disease between the earliest symptoms and the appearance of the rash or fever is the
   a. incubation period
   b. infectious period
   c. prodromal period
   d. stage one period

3. An infection acquired in a health-care facility during hospitalization is termed a(n)
   a. opportunistic infection.
   b. nosocomial infection.
   c. acquired infection.
   d. natural infection.

4. Patients with tuberculosis, varicella, and rubeola would require which type of infection precautions?
   a. large droplet infection precautions
   b. airborne infection precautions
   c. communicable disease precautions
   d. large droplet infection precautions

5. A circular, reddened area on the skin that is elevated and contains fluid is a
   a. vesicle
   b. pustule
   c. macule
   d. papule

6. If a vaccination series is interrupted,
   a. the series must start over.
   b. it continues without restarting the entire series.
   c. the age of the child determines if the series must be restarted.
   d. the child must rest six months before restarting the series.

7. STDs can be prevented through
   a. the use of a condom.
   b. the use of the oral contraceptives.
   c. abstinence.
   d. the use of vaginal sprays.

8. The incubation period for chickenpox is
   a. 1–2 weeks.
   b. 2–3 weeks.
   c. 3–4 weeks.
   d. 4–5 weeks.

9. In which type of isolation would a child with pertussis be placed?
   a. large droplet infection precautions
   b. airborne infection precautions
   c. communicable disease precautions
   d. large droplet infection precautions

10. The most important nursing action in preventing the spread of infection is
    a. the administration of antibiotics.
    b. placing all children in private rooms.
    c. good handwashing.
    d. good nutrition.

Student Name ______________________________

11. The primary risk related to rubella is
    a. exposure of a pregnant women.
    b. infection of lesions.
    c. high fever.
    d. exposure of immune-suppressed children.

12. Koplik spots in the mouth can be found in
    a. chickenpox.
    b. rubella.
    c. rubeola.
    d. mumps.

13. The risk of secondary infection in communicable diseases is reduced by
    a. giving all children antibiotics.
    b. keeping fingernails short.
    c. forcing fluids.
    d. isolating the child.

14. The disease that causes a "slapped cheek" appearance is
    a. Lyme disease.
    b. roseola.
    c. strep throat.
    d. fifth disease.

15. Chickenpox can be life-threatening to a child who
    a. is under six months of age.
    b. is immunocompromised.
    c. runs a high fever.
    d. contracts the disease a second time.

chapter **32**

The Child with an Emotional or Behavioral Condition

LEARNING ACTIVITIES

1. Match the terms in the left column with their definitions on the right (a–f).

_____ gateway substances	a. thoughts about suicide
_____ milieu therapy	b. attempt at a suicidal-type action that does not result in injury
_____ psychosomatic	c. action that is seriously intended to cause death
_____ suicidal attempt	d. physical and social environment
_____ suicidal gestures	e. common household products that can be abused to achieve an altered state of consciousness
_____ suicidal ideation	f. bodily dysfunctions that seem to have emotional and organic bases

2. List some of the psychologic disturbances seen in children who come from dysfunctional families.

   a. ______________________________

   b. ______________________________

   c. ______________________________

   d. ______________________________

3. List three signs of autism usually seen by one year of age.

   a. ______________________________

   b. ______________________________

   c. ______________________________

Student Name ______________________________

4. Manifestations of suicidal behavior include

   a. ______________________________

   b. ______________________________

   c. ______________________________

   d. ______________________________

   e. ______________________________

   f. ______________________________

5. Describe the treatment of autism.

   ____

   ____

   ____

6. What is the nurse's role when caring for a child with autism?

   ____

7. Describe the nurse's role in caring for a child with obsessive-compulsive disorder.

   ____

8. List five common signs and symptoms experienced by adolescents who are depressed.

   a. ______________________________

   b. ______________________________

   c. ______________________________

   d. ______________________________

   e. ______________________________

9. Give an example of a question the nurse might ask an adolescent suspected of being suicidal.

   ____

   ____

10. List three behaviors in adolescents that might point to an alcoholism problem.

   a. ______________________________

   b. ______________________________

   c. ______________________________

11. Give the four levels of substance abuse.

    a. ______________________

    b. ______________________

    c. ______________________

    d. ______________________

12. What are the two types of drug dependence?

    a. ______________________

    b. ______________________

13. List two strategies for the prevention of substance abuse.

    a. ______________________

    ____

    b. ______________________

    ____

14. List the four observations the nurse might make of children of alcoholics.

    a. ______________________

    b. ______________________

    c. ______________________

    d. ______________________

15. Give examples of each of the following clinical manifestations of a child with attention deficit hyperactivity disorder (ADHD).

    a. Inattention ______________________

    ____

    b. Impulsiveness ______________________

    ____

    c. Hyperactivity ______________________

    ____

Student Name ____________________

16. Describe the treatment of ADHD.

____

____

17. List five of the possible body changes associated with anorexia nervosa.

   a. ____________________

   b. ____________________

   c. ____________________

   d. ____________________

   e. ____________________

18. List some of the common behaviors of families of children with anorexia nervosa.
____

19. Describe the eating habits of a child with bulimia.
____________________.

THINKING CRITICALLY

1. In what way should care be altered when caring for a child with asthma who is also diagnosed as having ADHD?

OTHER LEARNING ACTIVITIES

1. Discuss in class how an adolescent suspected of being suicidal should be interviewed.

2. List two nursing diagnoses associated with depression. Discuss in a group how nursing care should be implemented for these diagnoses.

3. Care for a child who is admitted to the hospital with an emotional disorder.

REVIEW QUESTIONS

1. The risk of death increases in a suicidal adolescent when
   a. he is an only child.
   b. he has a learning disorder.
   c. he has a definite plan of action.
   d. his parents are divorced.

2. Alcohol is known to be a
   a. depressant.
   b. high source of protein.
   c. stimulant.
   d. antidepressant.

3. Marijuana has which of the following physical effects?
   a. bradycardia
   b. increased awareness
   c. anorexia
   d. tachycardia

4. The street name for a form of cocaine is
   a. crap.
   b. smack.
   c. hash.
   d. crack.

5. A side effect of using Ritalin may be
   a. nervousness.
   b. increased appetite.
   c. lethargy.
   d. weight gain.

6. Primary to prevention of substance abuse in children is a
   a. positive self-image.
   b. strong religious belief.
   c. strict family.
   d. good education.

7. Adolescents who seek help for a substance abuse problem usually do so because
   a. there are no other options.
   b. they have friends in treatment.
   c. they realize they need help.
   d. their family encourages them.

8. If a nurse suspects an adolescent is contemplating suicide, he/she should
   a. avoid the subject.
   b. ask the parents if they agree.
   c. ask the adolescent directly if he/she is thinking of killing him- or herself.
   d. observe him/her closely.

9. The best response to a depressed adolescent is
   a. "Cheer up, things will get better."
   b. "Let's talk about how you are feeling."
   c. "Things always seem worse than they are."
   d. "You are so lucky to have so many friends."

10. Children from dysfunctional families
    a. disassociate from their families.
    b. identify with parental values.
    c. long to be removed from the family.
    d. will not recreate the behaviors they have learned.

11. The type of drug dependence that causes withdrawal symptoms is called
    a. psychologic.
    b. pharmacologic.
    c. physical.
    d. mental.

12. Adolescents who drink even small amounts of alcohol are at increased risk to
    a. develop acne.
    b. become obese.
    c. have a drop in their intelligence.
    d. have an accident.

Student Name ______________________________

13. Bulimia is described as
    a. binge eating followed by self-induced vomiting.
    b. inability to eat due to fear of gaining weight.
    c. a systemic infection caused by a parasite.
    d. A secondary infection caused by a parasite.

14. Drugs used in the treatment of ADHD
    a. are addictive.
    b. inhibit the release of norepinephrine.
    c. may cause insomnia.
    d. are easily abused.

15. Antidepressants
    a. provide immediate relief of depression.
    b. should never be given to children under 12 years of age.
    c. must be taken three to four weeks before a therapeutic level is reached.
    d. can only be taken for short periods of time.

16. A 16-year-old male who has broken off with his girlfriend threatens to kill himself. The nurse knows that this behavior
    a. is attention-seeking.
    b. should be taken seriously.
    c. should be ignored.
    d. is a normal reaction to the situation.

17. The five-year-old child of parents who have recently divorced has started sucking her thumb. The nurse knows that this is
    a. a normal growth and development phase of many five-year-olds.
    b. cause for immediate psychiatric referral.
    c. response to the parent's separation.
    d. probably unrelated to the parent's divorce.

18. Children of alcoholic families
    a. do not usually exhibit any particular type of behavior.
    b. are often hyperactive.
    c. usually talk freely about the problem within their family.
    d. may bury their feelings.

19. ADHD is associated with
    a. learning disabilities.
    b. mental retardation.
    c. deafness.
    d. seizure disorders.

20. Children with ADHD
    a. may experience low self-esteem.
    b. are usually high achievers.
    c. usually have many friends.
    d. excel when given tasks that require intricate work.